ALLERGY IN CHILDREN

Allergy in Children

A Guide to Practical Management

Jan A Kuzemko, MD, FRCP, DCH

Consultant Children's Physician,
Peterborough
Clinical Teacher in Paediatrics,
University of Cambridge,
England

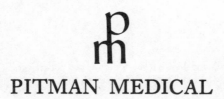

PITMAN MEDICAL

First published 1978

Catalogue Number 21 2031 81

Pitman Medical Publishing Co Ltd
PO Box 7, Tunbridge Wells,
Kent, TN1 1XH, England

Associated Companies

UNITED KINGDOM
Pitman Publishing Ltd, London
Focal Press Ltd, London

CANADA
Copp Clark Ltd, Toronto

USA
Fearon Pitman Publishers Inc, California
Focal Press Inc, New York

AUSTRALIA
Pitman Publishing Pty Ltd, Carlton

NEW ZEALAND
Pitman Publishing NZ Ltd, Wellington

British Library Cataloguing in Publication Data

Kuzemko, Jan Anthony
   Allergy in children
   1. Pediatric allergy
   I. Title
618.9′29′7   RJ386

   ISBN 0–272–79437–6

Text set in 11/12 pt Photon Imprint, printed by photolithography,
and bound in Great Britain at The Pitman Press, Bath

Contents

Preface   vi

1   Incidence and Genetic Aspects of Allergic Diseases   1

2   Causes of Allergy in Children   15

3   History and Examination   21

4   Food Allergy   27

5   Skin Allergy   41

6   Allergic Disease of the Upper Respiratory Tract   67

7   Ears   86

8   Asthma   91

9   Eyes   114

10   Allergic Reactions to Insect Bites and Stings   119

11   Drug Allergy   124

12   Allergy and Cystic Fibrosis   134

13   Allergy and the Nervous System   136

Index   139

Preface

One in every five children develops an allergic disorder sometime during childhood. Some conditions are short-lived causing little disturbance and family anxiety. Others, such as asthma, may be life-threatening. Skin problems may be responsible for many day or night hours of intense discomfort. A conductive deafness due to serous otitis media may present as unexpectedly poor school performance in a previously well-adjusted child. And yet much of such suffering is unnecessary and largely preventable.

This short text offers some guiding principles based on many years clinical practice of managing children with a variety of allergic conditions. Of necessity, here and there, an overlap occurs. This is intentional.

I am grateful to the many friends and colleagues for helpful discussions and comments and cherish especially the warm and yet poignant advice from the late Ronnie MacKeith. I am indebted to Mrs M Rushford, Librarian, Postgraduate Centre, Peterborough for help with references, to Mrs C Wilson for her tireless secretarial assistance, and Dr P Ryan, BA, for reading the manuscript through. Lastly I thank my wife for typing the many drafts and her courage, patience and understanding during the writing of this text.

Jan A Kuzemko

CHAPTER 1

Incidence and Genetic Aspects of Allergic Diseases

SMITH FIRST DESCRIBED anaphylactic reactions due to diphtheria antitoxin injections in guinea pigs in 1904.[1] This study paved the way for the observations of Von Pirquet and Schick[2] on serum sickness in man and their suggestion that such an altered reactivity should be termed *allergy*. Now the term is used interchangeably with hypersensitivity and can be defined as an abnormal and varied reaction which occurs in man following a contact with substances or agents which normally do not cause symptoms in other individuals. For instance, drinking cow's milk or eating eggs, fish, nuts, etc. does not produce any adverse effects in the majority of humans, but in a few, ingestion of any such foodstuff is followed within minutes by a series of characteristic symptoms and signs such as tissue swelling, urticaria or bronchospasm. Recently, the term *hypersensitiviness* has been introduced to mean a condition in which an immunological mechanism had been clearly shown. Neither of these terms should be confused with tolerance, which is a quantitative difference in the physiological response to any agent or substance. Thus, a small dose of a drug can produce significant pharmacological actions in one individual, whereas in another, much larger doses are required to produce a similar effect. The term *atopy* (Greek, meaning a strange disease) was coined by Coca and Cooke[3] who suggested that it should apply to those allergic diseases in man which appeared to have a familial or hereditary basis such as asthma, eczema, some skin conditions and migraine. Other conditions, for instance, the delayed tuberculin response or contact dermatitis were designated non-atopic states. Since then atopy has acquired many meanings. Some use it interchangeably with allergy and its disorders such as gastrointestinal allergy, tension fatigue syndromes in children, etc.[4,5] while others believe that the term should be restricted to those 'forms of immuno reactivity of the subject in which reaginic antibody (IgE) is produced in response to allergens in the environment'.[6,7]

1

There is little doubt that with the rapid advances in laboratory techniques in, for example, chemistry and immunology, some of the above concepts may have to be modified in the future.

The types of allergic reactions can be conveniently classified into four categories:[6]

Type I—Immediate hypersensitivity, anaphylactic

Allergens react with reagenic antibody (IgE) on the surface of basophils or mast cells and cause the release of vasoactive amines, e.g. histamine. The reactions occur within minutes of exposure to the allergen, e.g. pollenosis.

Type II—Cytotoxic

Allergens or haptens attached or associated with cell surfaces react with circulating antibodies. Complement, some mononuclear cells and other factors may be responsible for the cell damage. The reactions vary in the rapidity of onset, e.g. autoimmune haemolytic anaemia.

Type III—Arthus, antigen–antibody complexes

The reactions occur due to soluble toxic complexes, formed by combining precipitating antibodies with excess of antigens. The C_3 component of complement and neutrophil polymorphs are involved. The reactions take a few hours to develop, e.g. extrinsic allergic alveolitis due to *Micropolyspora faeni*.

Type IV—Delayed, cell mediated

The reactions are mediated by sensitised lymphocytes (thymus derived) which specifically combine with allergens. Lymphokines are released leading to inflammatory changes and infiltration of the site by lymphocytes and macrophages. The reactions require 24 hours or more to develop, e.g. contact dermatitis.

Allergy can affect most tissues of the body and result in a variety of clinical features which will vary as to their cause, pathophysiology and immunology. In addition, some authors are rather liberal in their use of the term *allergy*. For these reasons it is impossible to obtain exact figures of the incidence of allergic conditions in children.

In general it has been accepted that allergic diseases have an environmental and hereditary component. Some studies have shown that the environmental component is much more important than the hereditary one. The mode of inheritance remains unsettled and varies from multiple gene, single recessive to single dominant inheritance.[8,9]

Table 1.1

Country	Year	Condition	% affected	Source
U.S.A.	1960	Allergic rhinitis or asthma or eczema	19·54	Over 2,000 parents of children under 15 years were interviewed[10]
France	1964	Asthma Eczema Pollenosis Urticaria	4·2 11·4 11·06 14·75	Questionnaire study of 1,237 pairs of twins[11]
England	1967	Asthma Eczema (children only) Rhinitis Urticaria	3·1 3·6 11·4 6·9	Investigation into allergy in two general practices, taking the form of direct questioning and letters of enquiry[12]
Finland	1970	Asthma Pollenosis	2·1 2·7	Direct questioning and examination[13]
Sweden	1971	Asthma Eczema Urticaria Allergic rhinitis Contact dermatitis	3·8 2·0 2·6 14·8 4·8	Questionnaire study of 7,000 pairs of adult twins. These observations apply more correctly to allergy at all ages[8]
England	1974	Asthma Pollenosis Eczema	3·5 2·2 1·5	A retrospective record investigation into the incidence of allergic disease in an East London practice of 9,145. The percentage quoted gives over-all incidence, 80% were children with asthma and 7% children with pollenosis (5–15 years)[52]
England	1976	Asthma/wheezy bronchitis	*Male* 15·3 *Female* 7·0	A questionnaire and clinical study of 1,064 subjects under 16 years of age[76]
England	1976	Asthma Allergic and perennial rhinitis Urticaria Food allergy Gastro-intestinal allergy Eczema Others	4·9 8·2 5·7 1·6 0·8 1·2 0·6	Questionnaire study of 3,500 parents[41]

About 15–20 per cent of all children are affected by one of the major allergic disorders before they reach adolescence. The reported incidence from various countries is shown in Table 1.1.

The risk of allergy

The risks to a child of developing allergy are as follows:

Table 1.2

History of allergy	% risk
If both parents give positive history of allergy	30–40
If one parent gives positive history of allergy	20–30
If neither parent is known to have had allergy but a close relative has positive history	10–15
If there is negative family history	5–8
If there is negative family history but parents have one affected child with any major allergy	20–25

Compiled from various sources.[9,10,12,15,16]

Breast feeding and allergy

Kaufman and Crick,[17,18] found that if a baby was breast fed, and the mother, but not the father, had a positive history of allergy then the incidence of eczema was significantly less common than in those breast fed infants where both parents had a positive history of allergy. During the first two years of life, asthma developed in significantly fewer babies who were breast fed than in those who were bottle fed. A greater number of infants developed various types of allergies if they were born into families where both parents had an allergy. In general if both parents suffer from any major form of allergy, the onset of allergic disease in their child occurs much earlier than if one of the parents only gives a positive history of allergy. Thus, about 75 per cent of children will develop some form of allergy before the age of 4 years, if both parents are allergic, and about 50 per cent when only one parent is affected. About 40–50 per cent of subjects with eczema will subsequently develop asthma,[51,52] but the tendency to develop eczema during the first year or so of life appears to be less likely if the baby is completely breast fed during the first 3–5 months.[24,53,54]

It has also been shown that young babies may give positive skin sensitivity tests although they are symptom-free. It is not known whether breast feeding has a protective effect in such infants. We do know that there are protective factors in breast milk and some observations suggest that the infant who benefits most from breast feeding is one who has one parent with a negative allergic history.

It is likely that the development of allergy in children depends on many factors such as genetic predisposition, sex and month of birth, type of feeding and the child's environment. It is also suggested that strict breast feeding, or feeding with milk substitutes[25,26,110] and avoiding common potent allergic foods and agents during the first few months of life may lead to a reduction in, or even prevention of, some allergic disorders in children.

In a study of 58 babies born to allergic parents, Soothill *et al.*,[19-22] found that those infants who developed eczema or positive prick tests to a number of allergens had transient serum IgA deficiency during the period before symptoms developed. Further, the development of positive skin tests was related to the season of birth and to HLA AI B8 tissue antigens. In many babies the serum IgE was not raised. During the subsequent 12 months of observation, eczema cleared in some babies and skin tests became negative. These observations suggested that the production of allergy may occur in the very young baby whose mucus membranes may be exceptionally permeable to some antigens. In a further study of a small group of babies born to allergic parents, breast feeding and strict allergen avoidance resulted in significantly fewer instances of eczema at 6 months and 1 year of age than was found when such measures were not employed. In a Finnish study[23] of pollen and animal epithelium allergy, it was found that boys only were more likely to develop allergy if they were born during the months March, April and or September and October, although these findings were not confirmed by others.[24]

Nevertheless, all infants whether born into allergic families or not should be breast fed if at all possible for at least the first 3 to 6 months of life because breast milk contains specific antibodies such as immunoglobulin IgA which resist proteolytic digestion in the gastrointestinal tract and which may be of importance in preventing absorption of antigens from the baby's diet, thus reducing the risks of allergic reactions.[101-103] One must also say that despite the many recent studies, it has not yet been conclusively established that there is, in fact, a relationship between IgA deficiency, early exposure of the baby to environmental factors e.g. cow's milk and allergy.

Food allergy

It has been known for centuries that ingestion of certain foods such as cow's milk, eggs, fish or nuts can cause alarming reactions in certain individuals and that the removal of the offending substance leads to relief of symptoms. Although the subject still remains controversial and the true incidence of food allergy in the general population unknown, some useful information is appearing. For instance, it has been established that the Peyer's patches and lamina propria can generate immunological reactions and that the gastrointestinal tract contains plasma cells (IgA) and cells which are rich in IgG and IgM.[29–33]

For the purpose of simplicity, *food allergy* is defined as the development of unexpected reactions, not necessarily confined to the gastrointestinal tract, following ingestion of any type of food and *gastrointestinal allergy* as untoward reactions which primarily affect the alimentary tract. In this context, it is important to exclude *food intolerance* which is defined as the appearance of symptoms which occur following the eating of foods which some children have difficulty in digesting, e.g. vegetables, fruit.

Donnally[27] showed that a sensitising allergen can be passed in the mother's breast milk. A positive skin test reaction followed the injection of the breast milk whey of the mother who had eaten egg into a normal subject previously injected with the serum of a patient highly sensitive to egg white. He estimated that the egg white contained in the breast milk whey was present in an extremely minute amount, perhaps one part in a million, yet it was sufficient to induce a reaction. Donnally suggested that the normal intestinal mucosa might be permeable to certain food proteins which are then secreted into the breast milk of the mother and lead to sensitivity in the baby and subsequent development of clinical allergy. In this context it should be remembered that any medication taken by a nursing mother is excreted in her milk, e.g. antibiotics, antihistamines, narcotics, tranquillisers, thiazides, vitamins. Hence, any of these or other agents can be the cause of allergy in the baby.[104]

There is little doubt that hereditary predisposition plays a role in clinical manifestations of food allergy such as asthma, eczema and migraine, but the evidence that it does so in urticarial states, angioedema, allergic rhinitis and gastrointestinal allergy is less clear. Some children develop allergy to a specific foodstuff which not uncommonly is dominantly inherited.[28,38]

Any food can be allergenic, those most commonly encountered in paediatric practice comprise milk, egg white, chocolate, nuts, citrus fruits, fish, pork and tomatoes. Generally speaking, food allergy diminishes in frequency with age and this is especially so in children sensitive to egg white which is often associated with eczema or urticaria. Some believe[87] that juvenile polyps of the colon and nasal polyps are of allergic nature—and indeed the histology of both is similar.

Incidence

The exact incidence of food allergy in children remains unknown. Probably during the first year of life the prevalence rate of allergy, mostly to cow's milk proteins, is about 1 per cent of all infants born[34,35] and about 0·5 per cent throughout the rest of childhood.[36,37]

Gastro-intestinal allergy is at times a familial condition as has been well demonstrated by Gerrard *et al.*[38] who in a 10 year follow up of 150 children showed that about 17 per cent of the mothers of babies with cow's milk allergy had adverse reactions on testing with milk although they did not have clinical features. It has been observed also that if there is one baby in a family affected by cow's milk allergy, the chances are that one out of every two subsequent babies will be similarly affected.[39,40]

Allergic skin conditions

These can be divided into two groups: firstly, inflammatory conditions such as atopic dermatitis (eczema) and contact dermatitis, and secondly, urticaria and angioedema. Genetic factors are relevant in all allergic conditions with the exception of contact dermatitis where raised levels of serum IgE are not detected.[42-44] Children with active atopic skin conditions have raised serum IgE levels which return to normal a few months after the condition clinically subsides.[45] Many children also have increased levels of serum IgG,[46] the exception being those boys with the Wiskott–Aldrich Syndrome (a sex-linked recessive disease, associated with eczema, thrombocytopoenia and a tendency to serious infections and malignancies with a high death rate) where IgG levels are normal, IgE and IgA levels high, but where IgM antibody production is reduced.[47-50]

The true prevalence rate of allergic skin conditions in children is uncertain, because many parents and children do not recognise the significance of a rash and report it. This is especially so in cases of acute urticaria. In general about 5–8 per cent of children develop some kind of allergic dermatitis before they reach adolescence.[8,10,41,52] Eczema is a little less common than urticaria which is more common in girls. The incidence of urticaria in the total population is about 2 per cent and about 3 per cent in babies and children.[55-57] The rate increases if there is a previous history of asthma, eczema or pollenosis.

The nature of immunological disturbances in children with psoriasis is conflicting. Some authors have reported raised serum and salivary levels of IgA, serum IgG and in some raised levels of serum IgE.[42,43,107-109]

Hypersensitivity to drugs

In general, atopic children do not develop allergic reactions to drugs more often than normal children[58] though some studies suggest that penicillin hypersensitivity is common.[59,60,78] It has also been shown that subjects treated with two or more drugs at the same time are likely to develop sensitivities to all the drugs rather than to one only.[60] In many instances, however, it is difficult to distinguish an allergic drug reaction from idiosyncracy or toxic manifestations.[61-63] Sensitivity to aspirin is stated to be more common in subjects with asthma or rhinitis (2·4 per cent) and may be responsible for attacks of asthma or urticaria.[105] However, antibodies to aspirin have not been detected in sera of aspirin intolerant individuals and a suggestion has been made that prostaglandin PG_2 release may be inhibited.[106] For a concise review of adverse drug reactions, the reader should consult Amos.[111]

Occurrence of a new allergy in the child with an already active allergy

It is of interest that skin sensitivity tests to various allergens may give positive reactions in apparently normal subjects for months or even years before allergy or high serum IgE levels develop.[64,77,79,80] If these observations are confirmed the simple skin test may become a useful screening test. It is also true that some atopic children give positive reactions to some allergens which clinically do not appear to trouble them. For these reasons any data of the prevalence ratio of new allergies in the already allergic child are of necessity long-term clinical observations which do not give a true picture. Rackman[65] followed 688 asthmatic children whom he assessed after 20 years and observed that 17 developed pollenosis as adults although in 15 skin sensitivity tests were already positive when they attended as children. Ratner and Silverman[66] found that 59 per cent of children with eczema developed asthma and allergic rhinitis later on in life. In a study of 903 college students, 6 per cent who developed asthma had previously had allergic rhinitis.[70] In other studies the development of new allergies varied from 15 to 50 per cent.[54,67-69]

Similarly, an increased incidence of acute and chronic urticaria is found in those patients who have a family history of migraine,[71] some other evidence of atopy[72] or who themselves have previously had eczema, pollenosis or asthma,[71,73-75] although some clinicians dispute whether the history of atopy is relevant in patients with chronic urticaria.[56]

In an important study of 274 children who underwent adenoidectomy because of frequent episodes of acute otitis media, hearing loss and nasal obstruction, Kjellman et al.[81] found that a positive family history was often present, and that children had increased blood eosinophilia and raised serum IgE levels. This study supports earlier observations[82-84,86] and strongly suggests that before tonsils and adenoids are unceremoniously removed from children allergy should first be excluded, because a conservative approach to treatment may be of greater and more lasting value than elective surgery.[85]

Mortality and prognosis of allergic diseases in children

Deaths due to allergy are uncommon in children. About 25–35 children die each year from asthma in England and Wales[88] and occasional fatalities are reported from eczema vaccinatum,[89] cow's milk protein-allergy[90,91] and bee and wasp stings.[92] Some children die unnecessarily from the complications of treatment, especially long-term cor-ticosteroids,[93] over-use of xanthine derivatives and following anaphylac-tic reactions to antibiotics, especially penicillin.[94–96]

A 10 year study of allergy in a large group of children may be of interest.[97]

Table 1.3

Condition	Age of onset (%)			Remarks
	under 4	5–10	11–15	
Asthma	68·5	19·2	6·3	About 25% appear to have shown spontaneous clinical improvement during adolescence, outlook worse if they have had eczema or pollenosis. In a long term Swedish study[98] it was found that about 30% were symptom free. For details see Kuzemko[99]
Eczema	90	8·8	1·2	30% cleared within 3 years, another 15% in 5 years. The rest continue to have remissions and exacerbations. Outlook worse if they have asthma. Findings are in agreement with Musgrove and Morgan[100]
Pollenosis	28·1	32·2	39·7	About 14% had no relapses during 6 years of observation
Food allergy	99	1		Almost all settled within 3 years of diagnosis with the exception of egg white, fish and nut sensitivity
Urticaria	10	40	50	Penicillin often implicated. 95% acute, 5% chronic, i.e. symptoms persisting for 6–12 months

Allergy and surgery

Some controversy exists as to whether general anaesthesia and surgery during early life, e.g. Ramstedt's operation, predisposes to later development of respiratory tract allergy, such as asthma and hay fever. The reported studies are conflicting.[112-114]

Allergy and acute bronchiolitis in infancy

Until very recently it has been generally accepted that attacks of respiratory syncytial virus bronchiolitis in early infancy strongly predisposed to the development of asthma.[115,116] However, in a controlled study of 35 children it was shown that in 18 of the children minor episodes of bronchospasm occurred later on, but in such children symptoms disappeared by the age of 8 years. This study,[117] like the one previously published[118] suggests that bronchial hyper-reactivity may be inherited in a different way from atopy.

References

1. Smith, T. (1904) The degrees of susceptibility to diphtheria toxin among guinea pigs: Transmission to parents from offspring. *J. Med. Res.* (new series), **13**, 341.
2. Von Pirquet, C. and Schick, B. (1905) *Die Serum Krankheit.* Leipzig: Denticke.
3. Coca, A. F. and Cooke, R. A. (1923) On the classification of the phenomena of hypersensitiviness. *J. Immunol.*, **8**, 163.
4. Speer, F. (1954) Allergic tension-fatigue in children. *Annls Allergy*, **12**, 168.
5. Crook, W. G., Harrison, W. W., Crawford, S. E. and Emerson, B. S. (1961) Systemic manifestations due to allergy: report of fifty patients and a review of the literature on the subject (sometimes referred to as allergic toxemia and the allergic tension-fatigue syndrome). *Pediatrics*, **27**, 790.
6. Pepys, J. (1975) In: *Clinical Aspects of Immunology.* Ed. by Gell, P. G. H., Coombs, R. R. A. and Lachmann, P. J., 3rd ed., pp. 764‒779, 877‒902. Oxford: Blackwell Scientific.
7. Spector, S. L. and Farr, R. S. (1976) Atopy reconsidered. *Clin. Allergy*, **6**, 83.
8. Edfors-Lubs, M. L. (1971) Allergy in 7000 twin pairs. *Acta allerg.*, **26**, 249.
9. Edfors-Lubs, M. L. (1972) Empiric risks for genetic counselling in families with allergy. *J. Pediat.*, **80**, 26.
10. Rapaport, H. G., Appel, S. J. and Szarton, V. L. (1960) Incidence of allergy in a paediatric population: Pilot survey of 2169 children. *Annls Allergy*, **18**, 45.
11. Gedda, L. (1964) La complexe contribution du génotype à la prédisposition morbide. *Acta genet. Med.* (Roma), **13**, 321.
12. Leigh, D. and Marley, E. (1967) *Bronchial Asthma.* Oxford: Pergamon Press.
13. Alanko, K. (1970) Prevalence of asthma in a Finnish rural population. A study of symptomatic subjects tested for bronchial hyperreactivity. *Scand. J. resp. Dis.* suppl. 76, pp. 1–64.
14. Van Arsdel, P. P. and Motulsky, A. G. (1959) Frequency and hereditability of asthma and allergic rhinitis in college students. *Acta Genet.*, **9**, 101.
15. Bowen, R. (1953) Allergy in identical twins. *J. Allergy*, **24**, 236.
16. Hagy, G. W. and Settipane, G. A. (1969) Bronchial asthma, allergic rhinitis and allergy skin tests among college students. *J. Allergy*, **44**, 323.
17. Kaufman, H. S. (1972) Diet and heredity in infantile atopic dermatitis. *Archs. Dermatol.*, **105**, 400.

18. Kaufman, H. S. and Frick, O. L. (1976) Immunological development in infants of allergic parents. *Clin. Allergy*, **4**, 321.

19. Taylor, B., Norman, A. P., Orgel, H. A., Stokes, C. R., Turner, M. W. and Soothill, J. F. (1973) Transient IgA deficiency and pathogenesis of infantile atopy. *Lancet*, **II**, 111.

20. Stokes, C. R., Taylor, B. and Turner, M. W. (1974) Association of house dust and grass pollen allergies with specific IgA antibody deficiency. *Lancet*, **II**, 485.

21. Soothill, J. F. (1976) Some intrinsic and extrinsic factors predisposing to allergy. *Proc. R. Soc. Med.*, **69**, 6, 439.

22. Soothill, J. F., Stokes, C. R., Turner, M. W., Norman, A. P. and Taylor, B. (1976) Predisposing factors and the development of reaginic allergy in infancy. *Clin. Allergy*, **6**, 305.

23. Björkstén, F. and Suoniemi, I. (1976) Dependence of immediate hypersensitivity on the month of birth. *Clin. Allergy*, **6**, 165.

24. Pearson, D. J., Freed, D. L. and Taylor, G. (1977) Respiratory allergy and month of birth. *Clin. Allergy*, **7**, 29.

25. Glaser, J. and Johnstone, D. (1953) Prophylaxis of allergic disease in the newborn. *J. Am. med. Ass.*, **153**, 620.

26. Johnstone, D. and Dutton, A. (1966) Dietary prophylaxis of allergic disease in children. *New Eng. Med. J.*, **274**, 715.

27. Donnally, H. H. (1930) The question of elimination of foreign protein (egg white) in women's milk. *J. Immunol.*, **19**, 15.

28. Goldstein, G. B. and Heiner, D. C. (1970) Clinical and immunological perspectives in food sensitivity. A review. *J. Allergy*, **46**, 270.

29. Wright, R. and Truelove, S. C. (1966) Auto-immune reactions in ulcerative colitis. *Gut*, **7**, 32.

30. Hennes, A. R., Sevelius, H., Llewellyn, T., Woods, A. H., Joel, W. and Woolf, S. (1960) Experimental production of atrophic gastritis by a presumably immunologic mechanism. *J. Lab. Clin. Med.*, **56**, 826.

31. Katz, J., Kantor, F. S. and Herskovic, T. (1968) Intestinal antibodies to wheat fractions in coeliac disease. *Ann. intern. Med.*, **69**, 1149.

32. Kirsner, J. B. and Goldgraber, M. (1960) Hypersensitivity, autoimmunity and the digestive tract. *Gastroenterology*, **38**, 536.

33. Shiner, M., Ballard, J. and Smith, M. E. (1975) The small intestinal mucosa in cow's milk allergy. *Lancet*, **I**, 136.

34. Bachman, K. D. and Dees, S. C. (1957) Milk allergy. Observations on incidence and symptoms in well babies. *Pediatrics*, **20**, 393.

35. Freier, S. and Kletter, B. (1970) Milk allergy in infants and young children—current knowledge. *Clin. Pediatrics*, **9**, 449.

36. Bleumink, E. (1970) Food allergy: the chemical nature of the substances eliciting symptoms. *Wld. Rev. Nutr. Diet.*, **12**, 505.

37. Collins-Williams, C. (1962) Cow's milk allergy in infants and children. *Int. archs. Allergy appl. Immunol.*, **20**, 38.

38. Gerrard, J. W., Lubos, M. C., Hardy, L. W., Holmund, B. A. and Webster, D. (1967) Milk allergy: clinical picture and familial incidence. *Can. med. Ass. J.*, **97**, 780.

39. Despres, P., Plainfosse, B., Papiernik, M. and Sevinge, P. (1971) Les intolerances digestives aux protéines du lait de vache chez l'enfant. *Annls. Ped.*, **18**, 464.

40. Frier, S. (1974) In: *Clinical Immunology—Allergy in Paediatric Medicine*. Ed. by Brostoff, J., p. 108. Oxford: Blackwell Scientific.

41. Kuzemko, J. A. (1974) Unpublished observations.

42. Ogawa, M., Berger, P. A., MacIntyre, O. R., Clendenning, W. E. and Ishizaka, K. (1971) IgE in atopic dermatitis. *Archs. Dermatol.*, **103**, 575.

43. Clendenning, W. E., Clack, W. E., Ogawa, M. and Ishizaka, K. (1973) Serum IgE studies in atopic dermatitis. *J. invest. Dermatol.*, **61**, 233.

44. Gurevitch, A. W., Heiner, D. C. and Reisner, R. M. (1973) IgE in atopic dermatitis and other common dermatoses. *Archs. Dermatol.*, **107**, 712.

45. Varelzidis, A., Wilson, A. B., Meara, R. H. and Turk, J. L. (1966) Immunoglobulin levels in atopic eczema. *Brit. med. J.*, **II**, 925.
46. Juhlin, L., Johansson, G. O., Bennich, H., Hogman, C. and Thyresson, N. (1969) Immunoglobulin E in dermatoses: levels in atopic dermatitis and urticaria, *Arch. Dermatol*, **100**, 12.
47. Polmar, S. H., Lischner, H. W., Huang, U. N., Waldmann, A. and Terry, W. D. (1970) IgE levels in immunological states. *Clin. Res.*, **18**, 431.
48. Ammann, A. J. and Hong, R. (1971) Selective IgA deficiency. Presentation of 30 cases and a review of the literature. *Medicine*, **50**, 223.
49. Belohradsky, B. H., Finstad, J., Fudenberg, H. H. *et al.* (1974) Meeting report of the Second International Workshop on Primary Immunodeficiency Diseases in Man. *Clin. Immunol. Immunopathol.*, **2**, 281.
50. Fudenberg, H., Good, R. A., Goodman, H. C. *et al.* (1971) Primary immunodeficiencies—Report of a World Health Organisation Committee. *Pediatrics*, **47**, 927.
51. Perkin, J. M. (1972) Allergy in general practice. *The Practitioner*, **208**, 776.
52. Blair, H. (1974) The incidence of asthma, hay fever and infantile eczema in an East London Group Practice of 9145 patients. *Clin. Allergy*, **4**, 389.
53. Breast feeding: the immunological argument (1976) Editorial, *Br. med. J.*, **1**, 1167.
54. Blair, H. (1969) Aspects of asthma. *Proc. R. Soc. Med.*, **62**, 1008.
55. Bendkowski, B. (1968) Urticaria. *Curr. Med. Drugs*, **8**, 11.
56. Champion, R. H., Roberts, S. O. B., Carpenter, R. G. and Roger, J. H. (1969) Urticaria and angio-oedema—A review of 554 patients. *Br. J. Dermatol.*, **81**, 588.
57. Hellgren, L. (1972) The prevalence of urticaria in the total population. *Acta allerg.*, **27**, 236.
58. Steinber, R. H. and Levine, B. (1973) Prevalence of allergic diseases, penicillin hypersensitivity and aeroallergen hypersensitivity in various populations. Abstract 46, *Am. Acad. Allergy*, **51**, 100.
59. De Weck, A. L. (1971) Drug reactions. In: *Immunological Diseases*. Ed. by Samtor, M., 2nd ed., p. 425. Boston: Little Brown.
60. Levine, B. B. (1968) Immunochemical mechanisms of drug allergy. In: *Textbook of Immunopathology*. Ed. by Miescher, P. A. and Müller-Eberhard, H. J. Vol. 1, p. 271. New York: Graham-Stratton.
61. Lichtenstein, L. M. and Osler, A. G. (1964) Studies on the mechanisms of hypersensitivity phenomena. *J. exp. Med.*, **120**, 507.
62. Levine, B. B. and Zolor, D. M. (1969) Prediction of penicillin allergy by immunological tests. *J. Allergy Clin. Immunol.*, **43**, 231.
63. Russell, A. S. and Lessof, M. H. (1971) Hypersensitivity to drugs. *Clin. Allergy*, **1**, 179.
64. Hagy, G. W. and Settipane, G. A. (1971) Prognosis of positive allergy skin tests in an asymptomatic population. *J. Allergy Clin. Immunol.*, **48**, 200.
65. Rackman, F. (1952) Asthma in children. A follow-up of 688 patients after an interval of 20 years. *New Eng. Med. J.*, **246**, 815.
66. Ratner, B. and Silverman, D. A. (1953) Critical analysis of the hereditary concept of allergy. *J. Allergy*, **24**, 371.
67. Goodall, J. T. (1958) Asthma in general practice. *J. R. Coll. gen. Pract.*, **1**, 1.
68. Bono, J. and Levitt, P. (1964) The relationship of infantile atopic dermatitis to asthma and other respiratory allergic diseases. *Annls Allergy*, **22**, 72.
69. Novins, A. L. (1971) Atopic dermatitis. *Pediatr. Clin. N. Am.*, **18**, 802.
70. Hagy, G. W. and Settipane, G. A. (1976) Risks of developing asthma and allergic rhinitis: A 7 year follow-up of 903 college students. *J. Allergy Clin. Immunol.*, **58**, 330.
71. McKee, W. D. (1966) The incidence and familial occurrence of allergy. *J. Allergy*, **38**, 226.
72. Michaëlsson, G. (1969) Chronic urticaria. *Acta dermato-venereolog.*, **49**, 404.
73. Freeman, G. L. and Johnson, S. (1964) Allergic diseases in adolescents. *Am. J. Dis. Child.*, **107**, 549.

74. Green, G. R., Koelsche, G. A. and Kierland, R. R. (1965) Aetiology and pathogenesis of chronic urticaria. *Annls Allergy*, **23**, 30.
75. Hellgren, L. and Hersle, K. (1964) Acute and chronic urticaria. *Acta allerg.*, **19**, 406.
76. Davis, J. B. (1976) Asthma and wheezy bronchitis in children. Skin test reactivity in their parents and siblings. A controlled population study of sex differences. *Clin. Allergy*, **6**, 329.
77. Godfrey, R. C. and Griffiths, —. —. (1976) The prevalence of immediate positive skin tests to *Dermatophagoides pteronyssinus* and grass pollen in school children. *Clin. Allergy*, **6**, 79.
78. Rosh, M. S. and Shinefield, H. R. (1968) Penicillin antibodies in children. *Pediatrics*, **42**, 342.
79. Kjellman, N. I. (1976) Predictive value of high IgE levels in children. *Acta paediatr. Scand.*, **65**, 129.
80. Foucard, T. (1974) A follow-up study of children with asthmatoid bronchitis. Serum IgE and eosinophil counts in relation to clinical. *Acta paediatr. Scand.*, **63**, 129.
81. Kjellman, N. I., Synnerstad, B. and Hansson, L. O. (1976) Atopic allergy and immunoglobulins in children with adenoids and recurrent otitis media. *Acta paediatr. Scand.*, **65**, 593.
82. Koch, H. (1949) Allergy in the middle ear. *Progr. Allergy*, **11**, 134.
83. Miglets, A. (1973) The experimental production of allergic middle ear effusions. *Laryngoscope*, **83**, 1355.
84. Rapp, D. J. and Fahey, D. J. (1975) Allergy and chronic secretory otitis media. *Pediatr. Clin. N. Am.*, **22**, 259.
85. Wilson, W. H. (1971) Acute suppurative otitis media. A method for terminating recurrent episodes. *Laryngoscope*, **81**, 1401.
86. Lecks, H. I. (1961) Allergic aspects of serous otitis media in childhood. *N. Y. J. Med.*, **61**, 2737.
87. Alexander, R. H., Beckwith, J. B., Morgan, A. and Bill, A. H. (1970) Juvenile polyps of the colon and their relationship to allergy. *Am. J. Surg.*, **120**, 222.
88. Kuzemko, J. A. (1976) *Asthma in Children*, p. 9. Tunbridge Wells: Pitman Medical.
89. Copeman, P. W. M. and Wallace, H. J. (1964) Eczema vaccinatum. *Br. med. J.*, **2**, 906.
90. Stanfield, J. P. (1959) A review of cow's milk allergy in infancy. *Acta paediatr. Scand.*, **48**, 85.
91. Goldman, A. S., Anderson, D. W., Sellers, W. A., Seaperstein, S., Kniker, W. T. and Halpern, S. R. (1963) Milk allergy, skin testing of allergic and normal children with purified milk proteins. *Pediatrics*, **32**, 572.
92. *Registrar-General Statistical Review of England and Wales*, 1962–1971, Tables Pt. 1, Medical. London: H.M.S.O.
93. Fontana, V. J. (1970) Changing pattern of childhood asthma, steroid induced. *N. Y. J. Med.*, **70**, 1651.
94. Richards, W. and Patrick, T. R. (1965) Death from asthma in children. *Am. J. Dis. Child.*, **110**, 4.
95. Feinbger, S. M. (1961) Allergy from therapeutic products. *J. Am. Med. Ass.*, **178**, 815.
96. Wade, O. L. (1970) *Adverse Reactions to Drugs*. London: Heinemann.
97. Kuzemko, J. A. (1977) Children with allergy in Peterborough. Unpublished observations.
98. Kraepelien, S. (1964) Prognosis of asthma in childhood with special reference to pulmonary function and the value of specific hyposensitisation. *Acta paediatr. Scand. Suppl.*, **140**, 87.
99. Kuzemko, J. A. (1976) *Asthma in Children*, p. 9. Tunbridge Wells: Pitman Medical.
100. Musgrove, K. and Morgan, J. K. (1976) Infantile eczema. *Br. J. Dermatol.*, **95**, 365.
101. Goldman, A. S. and Smith, C. W. (1973) Host resistance factors in human milk. *J. Pediatr.*, **82**, 1082.
102. Walker, W. A. (1975) Antigen absorption from the small intestine and gastrointestinal disease. *Pediatr. Clin. N.Am.*, **22**, 731.

103. Gunther, M. (1975) The neonate's immunity gap, breast feeding and cot death. *Lancet*, **I**, 441.
104. Martin, E. W. (1971) *Hazards of Medication*, p. 279. Philadelphia: Lippincott.
105. Plummer, N. A., Hensby, C. N., Black, A. and Greaves, M. W. (1977) Prostaglandin activity in sustained inflammation of human skin before and after aspirin. *Clin. Sci. molec. Med.*, **52**, 615.
106. Szczeklik, A., Gryglewski, R. J. and Czeniawska-Mysik, G. (1975) Relationship of inhibition of prostaglandin biosynthesis by analgesics to asthma attacks in aspirin sensitive patients. *Br. med. J.*, **I**, 67.
107. Lai, A. Fat, R. F. and Van Furth (1974) Serum immunoglobulin levels in various skin diseases. *Clin. exp. Immunol.*, **17**, 129.
108. Oon, C. H., Goodwin, P. G., Kind, P. R. N., Sheah, P. P. and Fry, L. (1973) Salvary IgA in patients with psoriasis and dermatitis-herpetiformis. *Acta dermato-Venereolog.*, **53**, 340.
109. Guilhou, J. J., Clot, J., Meynadier, J. and Lapinski, H. (1976) Immunological aspects of psoriasis. *Br. J. Dermatol.*, **94**, 501.
110. Blair, H. (1977) Natural history of childhood asthma; twenty year follow-up. *Arch. dis. Child.*, **52**, 8, 613.
111. Amos, H. (1976) *Current Topics in Immunology, No. 5, Allergic Drug Reactions*. London: Edward Arnold.
112. Ballantine, T. V., Tapper, D., Mueller, H., Smith, R., Folkman, J. (1975) Pyloromyotomy. Does surgery in infancy increase allergy? *Pediatrics*, **56**, 404.
113. Collicott, P. E., Chappell, J. S. and Bill, A. H. (1972) Is there a correlation between allergy and infantile pyloric stenosis? *Pediatrics*, **49**, 768.
114. Johnstone, D. E., Roghmann, K. J. and Pless, I. B. (1975) Factors associated with the development of asthma and hay fever in children: The possible risks of hospitalization, surgery and anaesthesia. *Pediatrics*, **56**, 398.
115. Zweiman, B., Schoenwelter, W. F. and Hildreth, E. A. (1966) The relationship between bronchiolitis and allergic asthma. A prospective study with allergy evaluation. *J. Allergy*, **37**, 48.
116. Rooney, J. C. and Williams, H. E. (1971) The relationship between proved viral bronchiolitis and subsequent wheezing. *J. Pediatr.*, **79**, 744.
117. Sims, D. G., Downham, M. A. P. S., Gardner, P. S., Webb, J. K. G. and Weightman, D. (1978) Study of 8-year-old children with a history of respiratory syncytial virus bronchiolitis in infancy. *Br. med. J.*, **I**, 11.
118. McNichol, K. N. and Williams, H. E. (1973) Spectrum of asthma in children.—I. Clinical and physiological components. *Br. med. J.*, **IV**, 7.

CHAPTER 2

Causes of Allergy in Children

A CONSIDERABLE NUMBER of substances exist, usually proteins of some form, which are known to be involved in allergic reactions. Some are very obvious and common. However, in certain conditions the agents responsible for allergy appear to be obscure unless a very exacting history is obtained. It should be remembered that at times symptoms may be caused by similar or identical allergens which may be present in an animal or its products, e.g. cow's serum and cow's milk, horse serum and horse dander (cross reactions).

The following is a useful classification of antigens to which a child may become hypersensitive:

1. inhalants;
2. ingestants;
3. contanctants;
4. injectants;
5. physical agents;
6. miscellaneous.

Each of these categories is dealt with in detail in the text which follows.

Inhalants

In this group the allergen is absorbed through the mucous membrane of either the nose or the respiratory tract which acts as the shock organ. The concentration of skin sensitising antibody (IgE) in such tissues is relatively high. Hereditary factors appear to be of importance. Further, if in a particular child the shock organ happens to be elsewhere in the body, e.g. skin, the child may develop eczema or urticaria, but not rhinitis or asthma. The nature of antigenic substances is largely undetermined with the exception of ragweed pollen (antigen fraction E),[1-3] which is about 20 μ in diameter. Some pollen grains are considerably larger. Common allergens are pollens, moulds, animal danders (such as rabbit and cat), dog hairs, feathers, insecticides, and the house dust mites (*Der-*

matophagoides pteronyssinus or *farinae*). Common pollens include the grass plantain and tree pollens, especially the pollens of the birch, beech and oak. How pollen grains cause asthma is unknown. Theoretically they react with IgE antibody on mast cells in the bronchi causing the release of chemical mediators such as histamine, slow reacting substance, etc., leading to bronchoconstriction. Since the majority of pollen grains are too large to reach the small bronchi, it is possible that fractions of grain about 5 μ or so are responsible[7] or even a pollen extract.[8] It is also possible that there exists a reflex mechanism for which there is some evidence in man.[9] In general, pollens from brightly flowering plants are rarely associated with allergy in children because they are sticky and are carried by insects.

Animal epithelia

These are very potent allergens some of which are glycoproteins. Often a history of contact with horses or even wearing a dress which has been in contact with a horse may produce reactions. A crossed radio-immunoelectro-phoresis (CRIE) of allergen extracts of horse hair and dandruff using rabbit antibodies revealed 25 antigens, many of which were also identified in the serum[4] (thought to be a protein which immunologically is similar to serum albumin).[27] Cat dander is also important in children and it is especially useful to inquire about toys that the child may be playing with as some may have been stuffed with cat hair. Rabbit hair and guinea pig danders are also occasionally involved although animal hair is more often an irritant than a sensitiser. Dog epithelium is an extremely strong sensitiser[28,29] and sometimes a child may produce symptoms without the dog being in the room because there may be enough dander present on furniture or other objects. At least 25 per cent of subjects with asthma will give positive skin reactions to animal extracts.[30]

Bird feathers may act as sensitisers and although the active principle is unknown, there is evidence that the allergenic activity is contained in a keratinaceous protein mixture.[10]

House dust

Sensitivity to house dust is common because the dust contains a mixture of organic matter, dander, moulds, insects and pollens. Pure dust is probably just an irritant. The house dust mite (*Dermatophagoides pteronyssinus* or *farinae*) is a common sensitiser in children and associated with damp and humid conditions.[11, 12] Analysis of house dust by quantitative immunoelectrophoresis and crossed radio immunoelectrophoresis demonstrated 36 antigens.[5]

Cotton lint

These fibres are used in the manufacture of felt, upholstery and carpets. Cotton seeds are used in the production of oil and also are present in some fertilizers and animal feeds. There appears to be cross reaction between cotton seed and kapok as some children who are allergic to cotton seed may be found to be allergic to mustard and flax seed.

Orris root

This substance is used at times in the preparation of plasters and because of its odour it often forms the base for cosmetics.

Flax seed and kapok

Flax forms the basis for various products such as shampoo and kapok is also used in the manufacture of mattresses and toys. Linseed oil is prepared from flax seed and is used for furniture polish and varnishes and some hair sprays.

Moulds

Most of the common moulds involved are *Alternaria* and *Cladosporium*, which are found out-doors and grow on plants and some vegetable matter, and *Aspergillus* and Penicillin which are predominantly found indoors. The size of spores varies between 2μ in diameter for Penicillin to 5μ diameter for *Alternaria*. It is not known which part of the airway the spores have to reach to cause symptoms. Many moulds, especially *Aspergillus fumigatus*, the house dust mite and some bird feathers, not uncommonly are responsible for dual-asthmatic reactions, i.e. immediate reaction within a few minutes and a few hours later, a delayed-reaction. The subject has been fully reviewed by Pepys.[6]

Ingestants

Food allergens

The common allergenic foods in children are cow's milk, eggs, cereals, fish, nuts, spices, vegetables and fruit. Occasionally a child may become allergic to a food colouring which is used in the preparation of drinks or syrups.

Cow's milk proteins are important allergens in young children. At least 50 proteins have so far been identified of which beta-lactoglobulin is the commonest.[13-15] There is no beta-lactoglobulin in human milk.[16] Other identified proteins are casein alpha-lactalbumin, bovine serum albumin and bovine gammaglobulin. Boiling destroys some proteins, casein being the most resistant to destruction.

It is also important to realise that alpha-lactalbumin may be found in beef and other meat products, for example beefburgers and this too leads to allergy.

Allergy to eggs is widespread, as a rule it implies sensitivity to the egg white. It is doubtful if sensitivity to egg yolk exists. A child who is sensitive to chicken eggs will generally be sensitive to chicken meat, but there are exceptions. It is also useful to remember that boiling eggs will allow some of the antigen to be destroyed with the exception of the ova mucoid fraction.

At times it may not be clear that a child is sensitive to egg white, hence it should be remembered that eggs are constituents of various foodstuffs such as cakes, ice creams, mayonnaise, etc.

Lastly, certain vaccines are grown on chick embryos and should not be used in egg sensitive children.

Wheat is the most important allergen of the cereals. Wheat flour is used in the preparation of spaghetti, macaroni and also bread. I have not found rice or corn a common sensitiser in children.

Allergy to fish is not uncommon, and the history is usually self evident. The most extensive studies are those from Norway.[17] The majority of children who are sensitive to cod fish can tolerate cod liver oil.

Nuts are very strong sensitisers and are responsible for a variety of symptoms. They are widely distributed and used in confectionery. Reactions are usually severe and very specific, i.e. for a particular nut alone.

Vegetables and fruit may occasionally cause problems. Ripe tomatoes contain a glycoprotein. In orange juice and coffee beans the active agent is chlorgenic acid.

Contactants

The number of allergenic substances is limitless. Potential sensitisers in children are various antibiotics such as neomycin sulphate, ethylenediamine (used in the manufacture of rubber products, dyes, insecticides, oils, etc.), turpentine and benzocaine. Occasionally a child who is in contact with animal dander such as that of the cat or dog may develop atopic dermatitis, or likewise dermatitis may develop in a baby whose napkin has been washed in one of the proteolytic enzyme detergents.[18]

Injectants

In this category are included various drugs, although it should be remembered that drugs may be ingested or inhaled, and that immediate or delayed types of reaction may occur. Most commonly reactions occur following injections of foreign sera, e.g. anti-tetanic serum or allergy may develop to insect stings, or very occasionally to insulin.[24,25] Honey bee venom is known to contain at least five major allergens: hyaluronidase, phospholipase A,[20,21] melittin[19,22,26] and allergens B and C.[23]

Physical agents

These (e.g. cold, heat, sun, light) may be responsible for some of the cases of urticaria or angioedema.

Miscellaneous

Certain toothpastes or hand lotions may be found to contain Indian gum to which a child may be sensitive. A detailed history is most informative and important.

References

1. Ishizaka, K., Ishizaka, T., Lee, E. H. (1966) Physicochemical properties of reaginic antibody. *J. Allergy*, **37**, 336.
2. Henderson, L. L., Swedlund, H. A., Van Dellen, R. G., Marcoux, J. P., Carryer, H. M., Peters, G. A. and Gleich, G. J. (1971) Evaluation of IgE tests in an allergy practice. *J. Allergy Clin. Immunol.*, **48**, 361.
3. Bazaral, M., Orgel, H. A. and Hamburger, R. N. (1971) IgE levels in normal infants and mothers and an inheritance hypothesis. *J. Immunol.*, **107**, 794.
4. Lowenstein, H. and Weeke, B. (1977) Allergen characterization and isolation (horse hair and dandruff). *Allergolog. Immunopathol.*, **5**, 4, 318.
5. Carlsen, S., Lowenstein, H. and Weeke, B. (1977) Analysis of antigens and allergens in a commercial house dust (HD) extract by means of quantitative immunoelectrophresis (QIE) and crossed radio immunoelectrophoresis (CRIE). *Allergolog. Immunopathol.*, **5**, 4, 327.
6. Pepys, J. (1969) *Hypersensitivity Disease of the Lungs*. Monographs in Allergy, Vol. 4. New York: Karger.
7. Busse, W. W., Reed, C. E. and Hoehne, J. H. (1972) Where is the allergic reaction in ragweed asthma? *J. Allergy Clin. Immunol.*, **50**, 289.
8. Wilson, A. F., Novey, H. S., Berke, R. A., Sarprenant, E. L. (1973) Deposition of inhaled pollen and pollen extract in human airways. *New Eng. Med. J.*, **288**, 1056.
9. Widdicombe, J. G. (1977) Some experimental models of acute asthma. *J. R. Coll. Phys.*, **11**, 2, 141.
10. Berrens, L. (1971) *The Chemistry of Atopic Allergens*. Monographs in Allergy, Vol. 7, 104. New York: Karger.
11. Spieksma, F. T. (1970) Biological aspects of the house dust mite (*Dermatophagoides pteronyssinus*) in relation to house dust atopy. *Clinical exp. Immunol.*, **6**, 61.
12. Maunsell, K., Wraith, D. G. and Cunnington, A. M. (1968) Mites and house dust allergy in bronchial asthma. *Lancet*, **I**, 1267.
13. Bleumink, E. and Young, E. (1968) Identification of the atopic allergen in cow's milk. *Int. Arch. Allergy appl. Immunol.*, **34**, 5.
14. Goldman, A. S., Anderson, D. W., Sellers, W. A., Saperstein, S., Kniker, W. T. and Halpern, S. R. (1963) Milk Allergy. Oral challenge with milk and isolated milk proteins in allergic children. *Pediatrics*, **32**, 572.
15. Kletter, B., Gery, I., Freier, S., Noah, Z. and Davies, M. A. (1971) Immunoglobulin E antibodies to milk proteins. *Clin. Allergy*, **1**, 249.
16. Bell, K. and McKenzie, H. A. (1964) Beta-lactoglobulins. *Nature, Lond.*, **204**, 1275.
17. Aas, K. (1966) Studies of hypersensitivity to fish—A clinical study. *Int. Archs Allergy*, **29**, 346.

18. Gilson, J. C., Juniper, C. P., Martin, R. B. and Weill, H. (1976) Biological effects of proteolytic enzyme detergents. Symposium report. *Thorax*, **31**, 621.
19. Hoffman, D. R. and Shipman, W. H. (1975) Allergenic analysis of bee venom fractions. *J. Allergy Clin. Immunol.*, **55**, 73.
20. Sobotka, A. Franklin, R., Valentine, M., Adkinson, N. F. and Lichtenstein, L. M. (1974) Honey bee venom: Phospholipase A as the major allergen. *J. Allergy Clin. Immunol.*, **53**, 103.
21. Sobotka, A., Franklin, R., Adkinson, N. F., Valentine, M., Baer, H. and Lichtenstein, L. M. (1976) Allergy to insect stings—II. Phospholipase A: The major allergen in honey bee venom. *J. Allergy Clin. Immunol.*, **57**, 29.
22. Hoffman, D. R. and Shipman, W. H. (1976) Allergens in bee venom—I. Separation and identification of the major allergens. *J. Allergy Clin. Immunol.*, **58**, 551.
23. Hoffman, D. R., Shipman, W. H. and Babin, D. (1977) Allergens in been venom—II. Two new high molecular weight allergenic specificities. *J. Allergy Clin. Immunol.*, **59**, 147.
24. Hanauer, L. and Batson, J. M. (1961) Anaphylactic shock following insulin injection: Case report and review of the literature. *Diabetes*, **10**, 105.
25. deShazo, R. D., Levinson, A. I., Boehm, T., Evans, R. and Ward, G. (1977) Severe persistent biphasic local (immediate and late) skin reactions to insulin. *J. Allergy Clin. Immunol.*, **59**, 161.
26. Paull, B. R., Yunginger, J. W. and Gleich, G. J. (1977) Melittin. An allergen of honey bee venom. *J. Allergy Clin. Immunol.*, **59**, 334.
27. Stokes, C. R. and Turner, M. W. (1975) Isolation and characterization of cat allergens. *Clin. Allergy*, **5**, 241.
28. Varga, J. M. and Ceska, D. (1972) Characterisation of allergen extracts by polyacrylamide gel isoelectricfocusing and radioimmunosorbent allergen assay—II. Dog and cat allergens. *Int. Arch. Allergy appl. Immunol.*, **42**, 438.
29. Yman, L., Brandt, R. and Ponterius, G. (1973) Serum albumin—an important allergen in dog epithelia extracts. *Int. Arch. Allergy appl. Immunol.*, **44**, 358.
30. Frankland, A. W. (1967) Allergy to animals. *Acta Allerg.*, **22**, 175.

CHAPTER 3

History and Examination

History

The recognition of four aspects is essential if one is going to arrive at the correct diagnosis.

1. Detailed history is the single most important step.
2. A critical attitude should be adopted in interpreting the cause and effect.
3. The habit of keeping full records and notes is indispensable.
4. One must always remember that one is dealing with a growing individual and his family, hence it is important to adopt a comprehensive view.

General paediatric history should be obtained. Then detailed questions should be asked regarding possible allergy. It is always important to establish at what age the symptoms started, and to enquire as to their severity, recurrence and disappearance either spontaneously or following any specific treatment.

Child's environment

Specific questions should be asked about the onset of respiratory, nasal or eye symptoms; their associations with physical agents such as cold, winds, odours, e.g. tobacco, furniture polish, sprays or exposure to house dust. Enquiry should be made regarding any family pets such as dogs, cats, horses, birds, guinea pigs, etc., and it should be established whether symptoms are more common when the child has been playing with toys or playing outside the house. A careful note should be made of any behavioural or emotional problems as these may be relevant.

Enquiry should be made into the type of accommodation, whether old or new, the type of heating, and whether the house is fully carpeted. A full description of the child's bedroom should be obtained, with attention to such details as the presence of feathers, rugs and their types, woollen bedding or fluffy toys. This part of the history is often of great importance. A visit to the child's home by a Health Visitor may be most helpful.

Diet

It is important to obtain a full history with regard to breast or bottle feeding and the onset of any allergic disorder. At times it is useful to ask the mother to record for a period of one week or longer, all the foods which the child has been eating. This may give a clue to the diagnosis of urticaria. The effects of any food stuffs on the gastrointestinal tract should be noted and particular attention paid to the frequency and composition of the stools.

Effect of games and play

In a child suspected of asthma, one should ask directly whether prolonged exercise, that is of more than six to ten minutes duration, causes any wheeziness, cough or dyspnoea and how soon does the child recover from it. It should be remembered that exercise induced bronchoconstriction occurs maximally five to ten minutes after the exercise is completed and as a rule a child will fully recover following 20 minutes rest.

School attendance

The approximate number of days of absence from school each term should be noted. Confirmatory evidence is easily obtained by writing to a School Health Service Official.

Family history of allergy

This is of great relevance and should include direct and indirect questioning. Not uncommonly one finds that the child has an uncle with 'chronic bronchitis' who in fact has asthma or has a mother with 'chronic sinusitis' who in fact is suffering from allergic rhinitis. The history should be fairly extensive to include both sides of the family and should go as far back as possible. At times during the initial interview the parents will deny any history of allergy, but when asked to think about the subject carefully at home and write down accurately the family tree and possible diseases, it is surprising how revealing the picture becomes.

Social history

It is important to enquire about the occupation of the father and/or the mother and to establish whether anyone smokes in the house.

Immunisation procedures

A detailed history should be taken especially noting untoward reactions following injections.

Types of treatment

The use of any drugs and the child's response to them should be carefully noted. One should detail beneficial and adverse effects, daily dosage used and duration of treatment.

   Following such a general discussion about the child and his family, questioning should become specific depending on the chief complaint.

Gastrointestinal symptoms

Any history of vomiting and/or diarrhoea and its relation to feeds, should be carefully enquired into. Intestinal colic in the very young baby is sometimes observed as a symptom of gastrointestinal allergy. At times this is related to certain food stuffs of high sugar content which cause excessive fermentation in the small bowel, but most commonly the nature of the colic remains obscure. Allergy to cow's milk may on occasions mimic hypertrophic pyloric stenosis but the force of vomiting is less severe. In addition there will always be other signs suggesting the diagnosis of cow's milk protein intolerance. Clinical features associated with cow's milk protein intolerance can be very variable. As a rule there will be a history of recurrent vomiting and diarrhoea which may be watery, or stools which may be blood stained. Some babies fail to thrive and the diarrhoea becomes very severe resulting in generalised systemic and metabolic upset. Blood eosinophilia is commonly found in this group of babies. It is also worth remembering that some babies may be sensitive to the soy protein which is used in the treatment of cow's milk protein intolerance.

Skin

Specific questions should be asked regarding the areas of skin involved in the past and areas which have become involved fairly recently. It is important to make sure that the parent understands what eczema is, as I have seen babies whose dermatitis was due to scabies although the mother thought it was eczema. It is thus important to ask whether there is any associated itching and what specific treatment has been used in the past. Lesions which have recurred for a period of more than six months should be accepted as being of chronic nature.

Nose

Enquiries should be made as to whether there is any nasal discharge and if so whether it is purulent or watery and whether it is associated with mouth breathing, nasal obstruction or any non-specific upper respiratory tract infection. The age of the child may give a clue as to the possible cause. For instance, in the very young snuffly baby, food allergy should be considered whereas similar symptoms in the older child would suggest inhalant allergic or vasomotor rhinitis. Notes should be made about attacks of acute rhinitis, their severity and treatments used and their results. Occasionally a child with chronic sinusitis may present with headache, hence it is important to enquire carefully into its location, severity, duration, time of occurrence, i.e. by day or night, and any relation to other symptoms. Lastly a note should be made regarding any nasal or sinus operations and their results.

At this stage one should ask about any degree of deafness, aural discharge, tinnitus or pain. On occasions a child presenting with vertigo may be found to have an unhealthy upper respiratory tract rather than a neurological disease.

Respiratory system

Particular enquiry should be made regarding the presence of wheeze, whether this is of expiratory nature, and whether it is associated with any degree of shortness of breath. A history of 'recurrent colds' not uncommonly suggests an allergic basis. Specific questioning should be made about recurrent attacks of tonsillitis, otitis media, acute bronchiolitis or any slowly resolving chest infections. It is essential at this early stage to exclude cystic fibrosis. One should ask how often the symptoms recur and find out to what extent they interfere with school attendance, play activities and sleep. The child's health between episodes should also be enquired into.

Examination

Physical examination should be thorough and complete as in any child who presents for consultation.

One should keep an open mind and make absolutely certain that non-allergic conditions are not responsible for the child's symptoms. These should be suspected and completely excluded as errors of judgement may be made, e.g. a child with cystic fibrosis or $alpha_1$ antitrypsin deficiency may be treated as an asthmatic, or a child with chronic renal disease treated for recurrent angioedema.

It is therefore absolutely vital to consider the child as a whole, rather than to direct one's attention to the possible target organ of allergy. Nevertheless, certain features of examination should be stressed.

The child's face may give a clue to an allergic diagnosis. Discoloration and swelling beneath the lower eye lids (allergic shiners, bags under the eyes) is due to venous stasis produced by oedema of the mucous membranes which interferes with the venous drainage to the pterygoid plexus. There is also associated spasm of the muscle of Müller which is the only smooth muscle of the eyelid. Such a spasm will impede further the venous return both from the skin and the subcutaneous tissues. It is not known how long such features take to develop, but my impression is about 6 months. Typically these features are seen in children with perennial allergic rhinitis.

Careful inspection of the skin of the nose will often reveal a transverse nasal crease which is due to the tip of the nose being constantly rubbed backwards and upwards in order to relieve itching. Many such children will display facial grimaces such as wrinkling of the nose and mouth which helps them in relieving itching and nasal oedema. It is essential to examine the nose in detail and observe the colour of the mucosa, presence of secretions and any abnormalities such as greyish swelling of the inferior turbinates which is often seen in a child with allergic rhinitis. The presence of nasal polyps should be determined, as positive findings may give a strong clue to further investigations.

Mouth breathing is common in children with nasal allergy. Such children will often show high arch palates and occasionally chest deformities such as pectus excavatum. Children who have suffered with perennial allergic rhinitis for many years may develop dental malocclusion resulting from the oedema of the maxillary, nasal and paranasal cavities which interferes with venous drainage. This leads to hypoxic changes in the surrounding tissues and thus impairment of the efficiency of the muscles supporting the dental arch, allowing the tongue to push the incisor, molar and premolar teeth labially.

Although geographic tongue has been described in association with allergic diseases in children, I have seen it infrequently. Bald circumscribed patches occasionally appear on the side or tip of the tongue presenting a characteristic punched-out appearance. When in doubt about the appearance of the tongue, it is important to examine the other members of the family as congenital fissuring of the tongue is a familial condition occasionally encountered.

It has been stated that children with allergy often have long silky eyelashes. I am not entirely convinced that this is in fact so. Children with generalised eczema will often show a 'puckering' under the eyelids. Vernal conjunctivitis is occasionally seen in children and presents with intense itching, lacrimation and intensely red eyes. Diagnosis is straightforward provided the upper eyelid is carefully elevated and inspected. Inspection shows a mass of papules which resemble 'cobblestones' and a thick discharge which on examination contains an excess of eosinophils. The condition is often seasonal although food allergy may be implicated.

The mouth, throat and ears should be examined for any ulceration, tonsilar or adenoidal enlargement, serous otitis media and conductive deafness. Children with perennial allergic rhinitis often show a hyperaemic oropharynx and those with persistent post-nasal secretions may show hyperplastic lymphoid follicles of the posterior wall of the pharynx, which are possibly due to chronic irritation and infection.

The examination of the chest should determine any external abnormalities such as funnel or barrel chest, and the type of breathing and any associated bronchospasm should be noted.

It has been stated that allergic individuals have low systolic blood pressure. I have not been able to confirm this observation in children, nevertheless blood pressure should always be checked as a matter of routine.

The examination of the skin should be complete and diligent. The use of a magnifying glass is strongly recommended. In the baby the scalp should be examined for the presence of cradle cap and in older children hypopigmentation or loss of hair; the eyes should be examined for blepharitis and the ears for otitis externa. The examination should proceed downwards in an orderly fashion to determine whether lesions are of eczematous nature, or whether the skin is prone to dermographism. Pitting of nails is often associated with psoriasis and gentle stroking of the skin may produce whealing in urticaria pigmentosa (Darier's sign). When in doubt about the nature of a skin condition one should always seek the help of a dermatologist.

CHAPTER 4

Food Allergy

AS PREVIOUSLY STATED *food allergy* is defined as sensitivity due to foods affecting any part of the body and with the involvement of a definite immunological reaction; *gastrointestinal tract allergy* is similarly immunologically mediated but may be caused by foods, drugs, moulds and other substances.

Food allergy

Unquestionably food allergy has remained one of the most neglected areas in paediatrics largely because precise diagnosis is at times controversial, and because of the paucity of reliable confirmatory diagnostic tests. The reason for the diagnostic difficulties may be due to the change in antigenicity of foods as they are progressively digested in the gut and the large number of proteins which are present in foods, e.g. cow's milk alone contains at least 50 antigens. Undoubtedly the condition is over-diagnosed in North America where challenge tests with foods and elimination diet trials have been accepted as confirmatory evidence of allergy. At best such procedures offer only circumstantial evidence of sensitivity. Moreover there is no uniform agreement in literature as to what constitutes a challenge test—this is especially so when cow's milk is used.[6,13,106]

Incidence

The incidence of food allergy in infancy and childhood is unknown and varies from one part of the world to another depending on the type of food eaten in a particular country. In the infant about 85 per cent of allergies are associated with food; by the age of 4 to 5 years inhalants become of major importance.[33] The diet of a European child contains numerous chemical food additives, colouring matters, antibiotics and various food allergens. Reactions to foods have been estimated as being between 0·3 and 7 per cent throughout childhood.[1-3] Sensitivity to cow's milk proteins is stated to be present in about 1 per cent of all infants born.[4] In a detailed study of 2000 children in the southern United States, food allergy was found to be present in 6·6 per cent of the sample.[5] If there is one baby in a family affected by cow's milk protein allergy, the chances of subsequent siblings being affected are one in two.[7]

Pathogenesis

Broadly speaking three types of mechanisms may be involved in causing symptoms following ingestion of any food-stuff. These are shown in Table 4.1.

Table 4.1   Types of adverse food reactions

Immunological reactions:
Type I (IgE mediated)
Type III (Arthus)
Type IV (delayed sensitivity)
IgA deficiency states

Biochemical reactions:
Intestinal enzyme deficiencies, e.g. disaccharidase
Malabsorption S.
Tyramine headache

Unknown reactions to food contaminants:
Drugs e.g. penicillin
Azo dyes, e.g. jellies, jams, caramel, salad dressings, coloured toothpaste
Cyclamates
Contaminants, e.g. Aspergillus or yeast in cheeses, pickles, etc.
Fermented drinks
Other haptens

Immunological aspects

Prausnitz and Küstner[34] established convincingly that ingested dietary proteins could penetrate the intestinal mucosa, enter the blood stream and cause sensitivity reactions in the skin. We now know that the factor which mediates such a reaction is an immunoglobulin (reagin) IgE. Further studies have shown that as the child grows older this intestinal permeability to some protein antigens diminishes, although low levels of circulating antibodies can be detected throughout life. This suggests occasional and possibly minute amounts of protein absorption.[35,36] Supportive evidence was obtained from observations which demonstrated that in some children recovering from gastroenteritis, the mucosal permeability to some proteins actually increased, e.g. to egg albumin.[37] However, some animal studies also indicate that another mechanism may be operative, namely a defect in the immunoregulatory system involving IgE-suppressor T cells.[63]

Lymphoid tissue proliferation in the intestine and the infiltration of the mucosa with lymphocytes, plasma cells and eosinophils derived from blood occurs after birth most likely as an immunological reaction to ingested bacteria, foreign proteins, etc. since animals kept in a germ-free environment do not demonstrate such changes,[38,39] and when orally challenged with foreign protein, die of anaphylactic reactions.[40] These antibody producing cells contain an abundance of various immunoglobulins especially IgA and to a lesser extent IgG, IgM, practically no IgE and IgD.[42,43] In the newly born baby IgA is absent.[41] The function of the immunoglobulins in the gastrointestinal tract is to combine with proteins reducing or abolishing their antigenic properties.[44,45] The significance of polypeptides formed during digestion of proteins is unclear.[48] Although the secretory IgA differs from that found in the serum, there is evidence that it enters the blood stream and forms an important source of the circulatory IgA.[46,47] By the age 2 to 3 years the secretory IgA reaches almost adult levels.[41] It is suggested that in allergic children the secretory IgA activity is decreased, possibly due to a mucosal defect.[44,49]

IgE forming plasma cells in the mucosa and the reaginic antibody produced react with food allergens on the surface of mast cells or basophils triggering a biochemical chain reaction and leading to the release of histamine, kinins and slow-reacting substance and other vasoactive agents.[50-52] Although IgE does not cross the placenta evidence exists of the presence of specific IgE antibody during the first 24 hours of life.[53,54]

IgE mediated reactions to food (Type I) are the most common in children and occur within minutes of ingestion of a particular dietary protein and may cause a variety of symptoms such as the swelling of lips, mouth, urticaria, gastrointestinal upset or breathing difficulties. Diagnosis is usually straightforward.

Some children develop symptoms a few hours after ingestion of a food. It has not been convincingly established that these reactions are associated with the Type III (toxic complex) or Type IV (cellular hypersensitivity) mechanisms,[31,33,99] although there is evidence that some babies allergic to cow's milk may show such reactions.[55,56]

Clinical manifestations

The variety of features attributed to allergy to foods are summarised in Table 4.2.

The most common foods responsible for sensitivity reactions in infants and children are:

cow's milk;   eggs (as a rule egg white);
wheat;   chocolate;

cheese;
fish (salt water and fresh water);
shellfish (especially cockles and lobsters);
chicken meat;
nuts;
vegetables;

fruits (especially tomatoes, pineapples and strawberries);
mushrooms;
yeasts;
spices and seasonings;
food additives;
drugs.

Foods that are rarely allergenic are:

rice;
lamb;
vegetables (e.g. lettuce);

fruits (e.g. apples);
gelatin.

Table 4.2

Gastrointestinal features:
Mouth ulcers,[8] geographical tongue,[9] intestinal colic,[18,19] spasm of pylorus,[18,19] diarrhoea and vomiting,[27,108] haematemesis,[27] dyspepsia,[29] colitis[10]

Skin:
Urticaria,[20] eczema,[27,108] angioedema[21]

Respiratory system:
Rhinitis,[27] asthma,[27,108] serous otitis media[26]

Central nervous system:
Headache,[11] irritability,[11] tension fatigue[15,16]

Blood:
Iron deficiency anaemia,[24] Heiner's syndrome[12]

Kidney:
Haematuria,[17] albuminuria,[28,30] enuresis[14]

Other:
Anaphylaxis,[27,28] recurrent fever,[29] infantile cortical hyperostosis,[13] recurrent joint swellings,[29] cot death,[22,23] failure to thrive and oedema[32]

Diagnosis

The diagnosis of food allergy depends on obtaining an accurate history, a carefully kept food diary, confirmatory investigations and a clinical trial of eliminating the suspected food and subsequently obtaining a positive challenge with that particular food. With the exception of children with gastrointestinal allergy physical examination is usually negative. A scheme for investigation of a baby with suspected cow's milk allergy is shown below:

A scheme for investigation of a baby with suspected cow's milk allergy

1. Admission to hospital

2. Routine studies:

       a. full and differential blood count; if iron deficiency anaemia—serum iron and binding capacity;
       b. sweat test to exclude cystic fibrosis;
       c. skin tests, RAST and PRIST;
       d. serum immunoglobulins;
       e. stools for pH sugar, blood and eosinophils;
       f. peroral jejunal biopsy for histology and enzyme studies;
       g. duodenal juice for giardia lamblia, bacteriology and precipitating antibodies

3. Challenge test with cow's milk (see text)

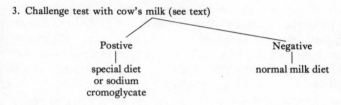

Postive	Negative
special diet or sodium cromoglycate	normal milk diet

4. Review weekly

Skin sensitivity tests

It should be stated that a positive (prick) skin test to a particular antigen does not indicate that a particular food causes symptoms. In general when any food causes anaphylactic reactions skin sensitivity tests will be positive. In some children positive tests may be obtained to foods not previously suspected by history. Such positive reactions should be interpreted with caution as a restrictive elimination diet trial may cause more harm than good.

There is no place in diagnosing food allergy by the intracutaneous injection of dilutions of food extracts in order to reproduce symptoms and signs, or by administration of such extracts sublingually.[25,57,95] The reactions obtained are variable, non-specific and may be alarming.

Although skin tests have a limited value in diagnosis of food allergy, they should be performed to confirm the clinical history and in those children who may be sensitive to egg or chicken meat. This is as a precaution against anaphylactic reactions which may occur when vaccines containing egg are used. Such children should be skin tested with a vaccine diluted to 1:100 with saline. If a negative test is obtained it is quite safe to proceed with the vaccination.

Radioallergosorbent test (RAST) or paper radio immunosorbent test (PRIST)

These tests detect specific and serum IgE antibodies. If it is remembered that some non-atopic and asymptomatic infants may give positive results, it is a useful adjunct in the diagnosis of IgE mediated food allergy and correlates well with clinical history.[58-60,109] The highest levels of specific IgE to foods are obtained in children with active eczema, and those with a past history of eczema, and the lowest levels in those who suffer from urticaria.[61,62]

Treatment

The essence of management is to avoid a particular food responsible for clinical symptoms. At all times the adequacy of any diet should be discussed with a dietitian to ensure a full intake of proteins, carbohydrates, vitamins and minerals, especially when any milk substitute formulas are used. The progress of the child should be periodically reviewed and very small amounts of the offending food added from time to time to the diet. The majority of children will be able to tolerate the offending food in 6 to 12 months but some cannot for many years.

We find oral hyposensitisation with foods of no benefit in children.

In certain situations where food allergy is strongly suspected but definite evidence is lacking, an elimination diet should be tried. We find it particularly useful in children with chronic urticaria. Table 4.3 shows the diet and scheme we use:

Instructions

Make sure foods are cooked well (cooking reduces antigenicity of some foods). Keep to the diet for 14 days. After 14 days introduce one food every 7 days from the forbidden list. Keep an accurate food diary and record of symptoms.

At times following such a scheme, sensitivity to unidentified food is lost, but the re-introduction of a normal diet causes symptoms. Depending on the severity of the condition, it is worth persisting with a modified diet blindly for from 2 to 4 months as the results can be quite rewarding.

For a full practical list of milk free and egg free diets, etc., the reader is referred to *Diets for Sick Children* by Francis and Dixon.[67]

Gastrointestinal tract allergy

Allergic reactions within the gastrointestinal tract may be caused by foods, food contaminants which may act as haptens, inhalants, moulds and drugs such as penicillin, causing bowel disturbance such as diarrhoea, vomiting, abdominal pains, oedema of the lips and palate or malabsorption. However, concomitant extra-gastrointestinal reactions may also occur.

Cow's milk sensitivity, of major importance in the very young, has

Table 4.3 Elimination diet

Foods allowed	Foods not allowed
Rice Rice flour	Flour and its products, e.g. bread, cakes, biscuits

Meat:
    lamb
    beef
    bacon
	Meat:
	    pork

	Fish and sea foods
Margarine Olive and corn oils Sun flower seed oil	Milk and milk products, e.g. butter, cheese, chocolate

Fruits:
    lemons
    grapefruit
    pineapples
    prunes
    apricots (jam)
	Fruits:
	    tomatoes
	    oranges
	    strawberries
	    nuts

Vegetables:
    carrots
    lettuce
    potatoes
	Vegetables:
	    beans
	    peas

Salt Sugar Vinegar	Soft drinks Sweets Tea Coffee
(No medicines allowed at any time)	

From various sources.[64-66]

been the most fully studied condition although definitive diagnosis is still difficult. Immunological reactions occur in other gastrointestinal diseases of childhood, such as gluten-induced enteropathy[68,69] Crohn's disease[70] and ulcerative colitis,[71] but the relationship of those conditions to allergy remains undecided.

Cow's milk sensitivity in infants

Incidence of this condition is under 1 per cent of all infants. Boys appear to be affected twice as commonly as girls. If one baby has the condition, the chances in subsequent siblings are 1 in 2.

Clinical manifestations. Two types of presentations are seen:

a. The baby presents within the first 3 months of life with recurrent vomiting, diarrhoea and intestinal colic. The stools are often watery and contain very small amounts of fresh blood. Some babies develop malabsorption, iron deficiency anaemia and fail to gain weight adequately. Rarely, functional intestinal obstruction develops or persistent severe diarrhoea occurs which may lead to serious metabolic complications and occasionally death.

b. The baby is usually older, between 6 and 18 months of age, and has intermittent periods of vomiting and diarrhoea, and occasional peripheral oedema which is due to protein-losing enteropathy. Blood and/or stool eosinophilia may be noted.

In both presentations there may be eczema or respiratory symptoms. Anaphylactic shock causing death has been described,[6,10,72] but clear cut evidence of its existence is lacking. If a baby with an absent radius and thrombocytopoenia develops diarrhoea, cow's milk allergy should be strongly suspected.[80,81]

Similar clinical and histological features may occur due to soy milk protein,[73-76] which is used by some to treat cow's milk sensitivity.

Pathogenesis. Cow's milk contains at least 50 antigens, of which five have been fully identified—beta-lactoglobulin, casein, alpha-lactalbumin, bovine serum albumin and bovine gammaglobulin. Beta-lactoglobulin sensitivity is numerically the most common, and has been shown to produce immunological reactions consistently.[62,77-79] It is also known that mild or very severe enteropathy simulating coeliac disease may develop, but the exact nature of mucosal cell damage is as yet unknown. As stated earlier Type I, Type III and Type IV (Coombs and Gell classification) reactions have been described in this condition.

Diagnosis. When a doctor suspects cow's milk allergy, he should discontinue cow's milk and replace it by a milk substitute. Symptoms should abate within 24 to 48 hours. After 2 to 4 days, 5 ml of cow's milk should be given orally. If there is no reaction within 4 hours, 10 ml of cow's milk should be given with every meal and the dose increased by 5 ml with each feed every day. After 5 days, normal milk feeds should be offered. The absence of symptoms (bulky stools or blood in stools and poor weight gain) within 30 days is considered a negative test (modified after[6,83,84]).

However, such a challenge test does not distinguish between cow's milk allergy and lactose intolerance—indeed these two conditions may co-exist.[82] Many doctors believe that no further investigations should be performed at this stage and it is sufficient to carry on with a milk substitute for the next 6 to 12 months and then re-challenge with cow's milk.[107]

My view is that a small intestinal biopsy should be performed early as it will demonstrate any histological changes in the mucosa and biochemical studies will determine the presence or absence of any disaccharidases. Histological changes are non-specific, varying from minor villous abnormality to subtotal villous atrophy.[84] [86] Others believe that two jejunal biopsies should be done—the first before an antigenic challenge with cow's milk and the second afterwards and evidence of an immunological reaction sought.[79,87,88] It is doubtful if such a procedure will be widely accepted. Immunological studies of duodenal juices may be of value[86] and the lymphoblast transformation test may become of further use in early diagnosis.[96]

Treatment. Milk substitute should be used for 6 to 12 months before cow's milk is introduced again. The majority of babies will be able to tolerate cow's milk after that period. Failure to thrive at any stage calls for a full re-investigation to exclude gluten-induced enteropathy, transient wheat, gluten or soy protein intolerance and other conditions. Types of milk, milk substitutes and foods currently employed in treatment are shown in Table 4.4.

Sodium cromoglycate

There is clinical evidence that the prophylactic administration of pure sodium cromoglycate may be of value in immunologically mediated gastrointestinal tract diseases such as cow's milk protein allergy,[78,89,90] ulcerative colitis,[91] chronic proctitis,[92] gastritis varioliformis[93] and diarrhoea associated with mastocytosis.[94] There is also clinical evidence that children with food allergies to eggs, fish, fruits, nuts, vegetables, chocolate, penicillin and some dyes may derive benefit from oral sodium cromoglycate,[97,98,101] especially those whose reactions to foods are IgE mediated.

The mode and site of action of sodium cromoglycate in the gut is unknown but the pharmacokinetics[100] of sodium cromoglycate would

Table 4.4

Cow's milk alternatives	Remarks
Milk:	
Human	Best, can be bought commercially from some hospitals, expensive
Goat	Occasionally successful but cross reactivity with cow's milk protein may occur
Allergilac	Cow's milk preparation from which most lactalbumin and soluble proteins have been removed, contains lactose
Milk substitutes:	
Nutramigen	Hydrolysed protein milk containing casein; sugar is sucrose, most popular
Pregestimil	Hydrolysed casein, contains glucose
Velactin	Soy protein, sugar is glucose
Prosobee (liquid)	Soy protein, sugar is glucose
Sobee (powder)	Soy protein, sugar is sucrose
Other:	
Meat products, e.g. comminuted chicken meat	Essential to add sugars, fats and vitamins, see Westall.[102]
Vivonex	Crystalline pure amino-acid mixture, containing glucose, animal fat and minerals. Occasionally useful in the early stages of treatment. For details see Beigler,[103] Belin,[104] Hyman et al.[105]

strongly suggest a local stabilising effect on the sensitised mast cells in the mucosa.

The dose of oral sodium cromoglycate in the treatment of food allergy varies between 50 mg before each feed to 100 mg before meals in older children. Treatment should be continued for 4 to 6 months before food challenge is performed. The results, especially in cow's milk allergy, are encouraging and no side-effects of oral cromoglycate treatment have so far been described.

References

1. Bachman, K. D. and Dees, S. C. (1957) Milk allergy. Observations on incidence in well babies. *Pediatrics,* **20,** 393.
2. Goldstein, G. B. and Heiner, D. C. (1970) Clinical and immunological perspectives in food sensitivity. *J. Allergy,* **46,** 270.

3. Ament, M. E. (1972) Malabsorption syndromes in infancy and childhood. *J. Pediatr.*, **81**, 685, 867.
4. Freier, S. and Kletter, B. (1970) Milk allergy in infants and young children. *Clin. Pediatrics*, **9**, 49.
5. Arbeiter, H. I. (1967) How prevalent is allergy among United States schoolchildren? *Clin. Pediatrics*, **6**, 140.
6. Goldman, A. S., Anderson, D. W., Sellers, W. A., Saperstein, S., Kniker, W. T. and Halpern, S. R. (1963) Milk allergy—I. Oral challenge with milk and isolated milk proteins in allergic children. *Pediatrics*, **32**, 425.
7. Despres, P., Plainfosse, B., Papiernik, M. and Sevinge, P. (1971) Les intolerances digestives aux protéines dulait de vache chez l'enfant. *Ann Ped.*, **18**, 464.
8. Glaser, J. (1956) *Allergy in Childhood*, pp. 84–86. Springfield: Charles C. Thomas.
9. McLendon, P. A. and Jaeger, D. S. (1953) Milk intolerance, the cause of a nutritional entity: A clinical study. *South Med. J.*, **36**, 571.
10. Gryboski, J. D. (1967) Gastrointestinal milk allergy in infants. *Pediatrics*, **40**, 354.
11. Unger, L. and Unger, A. H. (1952) Headaches of allergic origin. *J. Allergy*, **23**, 429.
12. Heiner, D. C., Sears, J. W. and Kniker, W. T. (1962) Multiple precipitins to cow's milk in chronic respiratory disease, including poor growth, gastrointestinal symptoms, evidence of allergy, iron deficiency anaemia and pulmonary hemosiderosis. A Syndrome. *Amer. J. Dis. Child.*, **103**, 634.
13. Bowman, R. E., Piston, R. W. and Meeks, E. A. (1966) Infantile cortical hyperostosis: an allergic disease? *S. med. J.*, **59**, 795.
14. Ammann, P. and Rossi, E. (1966) Allergic haematuria. *Arch. dis. Child.*, **41**, 539.
15. Speer, F. (1958) The allergic tension-fatigue syndrome in children. *Int. archs Allergy*, **12**, 207.
16. Crook, W. G. (1975) Food allergy—The great masquerader. *Pediatr. Clin. N. Am.*, **22**, 227.
17. Breneman, J. C. (1959) Allergic cystitis: the cause of nocturnal enuresis. *Gen. Practn.*, **20**, 84.
18. Deamer, W. C. (1973) Recurrent abdominal pain. *Pediatrics*, **51**, 307.
19. Crook, W. G. (1970) Recurrent abdominal pain. *Pediatrics*, **46**, 969.
20. Halpern, S. R. (1965) Chronic hives in children. An analysis of 75 cases. *Annls Allergy*, **23**, 589.
21. Champion, R. H. (1970) Urticaria and angioedema. *Brit. J. hosp. Med.*, **3**, 233.
22. Parish, W. E., Barrett, A. M., Coombs, R. R. A., Gunther, M. and Camps, E. (1960) Hypersensitivity to milk and sudden death in infancy. *Lancet*, **I**, 1106.
23. Gold, E. I. and Adelson, L. (1964) The role of antibody to cow's milk proteins in sudden death syndrome. *Pediatrics*, **33**, 541.
24. Wilson, J. F. (1964) Milk induced gastrointestinal bleeding in infants with hypochronic microcytic anaemia. *J. Am. med. Ass.*, **189**, 7, 568.
25. Breneman, J. C. (1974) Final report of the food allergy committee of the American College of Allergists on the clinical evaluation of sublingual provocative testing method for diagnosis of food allergy. *Annls Allergy*, **33**, 164.
26. Chan, J. C. M., Logan, G. B. and McBean, J. B. (1967) Serous otitis media and allergy. *Am. J. Dis. Child.*, **114**, 684.
27. Golbert, T. M. (1972) Food allergy and immunologic diseases of the gastrointestinal tract. In: *Allergic Diseases—Diagnosis and Management*. Ed. by Patterson, R. Philadelphia: Lippincott.
28. Crook, W. G. (1972) Genitourinary allergy. In: *Allergy and Immunology in Children*. Ed. by Speer, F., Dockhorn, R. J. and Shira, J. E., p. 692. Springfield: Charles C. Thomas.
29. Roy, C. and Dubois, R. (1973) Gastroenterologic disorders. In: *Immunologic Disorder in Infants and Children*. Ed. by Stiehm, R. E. and Fulgniti, V. A., 1st ed., p. 382. Philadelphia: Saunders.
30. Matsumura, T., Kuroume, T. and Fukushima, I. (1966) Significance of food allergy in the aetiology of orthostatic albuminuria. *J. asthma Res.*, **3**, 325.

31. Gell, P. G. H., Coombs, R. R. A. and Lachmann, P. J. (1975) Clinical Aspects of Immunology. 3rd ed., pp. 761–779. Oxford: Blackwell Scientific.
32. Waldmann, T. A., Wochner, R. D., Laster, L. and Gordon, R. S. (1967) Allergic gastroenterapathy. *New. Eng. Med. J.*, **276**, 761.
33. Marger, J. (1970) Food allergies. *Postgrad. Med.*, 230.
34. Prausnitz, C. and Küstner, H. (1921) Studies on supersensitivity. Cbl Bakteriol., **86**, 160.
35. Gunther, M., Cheek, R., Matthews, R. H. and Coombs, R. R. A. (1962) Immune responses to cow's milk proteins taken by mouth. *Int. archs Allergy*, **21**, 257.
36. Wright, R., Taylor, K. B., Truelove, S. C. and Aschaffenburg, R. (1962) Circulating antibodies to cow's milk proteins and gluten in the newborn. *Br. med. J.*, **II**, 513.
37. Gruskay, F. L. and Cooke, E. (1955) The gastrointestinal absorption of unaltered protein in normal infants and in infants recovering from diarrhoea. *Pediatrics*, **40**, 354.
38. Thorbecke, G. J. (1959) Some histological and functional aspects of lymphoid tissue in germ-free animals. *Ann. N.Y. Acad. Sci.*, **78**, 237.
39. Gowans, J. L. and Knight, E. J. (1964) The route of re-circulation of lymphocytes in the rat. *Proc. R. Soc.*, **B 159**, 257.
40. Coates, M. E. and O'Donoghue, P. H. (1967) Milk allergy in infant germ-free rabbits. *Nature, Lond.*, **21**, 3, 307.
41. Sahvilati, E. (1972) Immunoglobulin containing cells in the intestinal mucosa and immunoglobulins in the intestinal juice in children. *Clinical exp. Immunol.*, **2**, 415.
42. Crabbe, P. A. and Heremans, J. F. (1966) The distribution of immunoglobulin containing cells along the gastrointestinal tract. *Gastroenterology*, **51**, 305.
43. Ishizaka, K. and Ishizaka, T. (1970) Biological function of γE antibodies and mechanisms of reaginic hypersensitivity. *Clin. exp. Immunol.*, **6**, 25.
44. Tomasi, T. B. and Katz, L. (1971) Human antibodies against bovine immunoglobulin M in IgA deficient sera. *Clin. exp. Immunol.*, **9**, 3.
45. Walker, W. A. (1976) Host defence mechanisms in the gastrointestinal tract. *Pediatrics*, **57**, 901.
46. Bull, D. M., Bienenstock, J. and Tomasi, T. B. (1971) Studies on human intestinal immunoglobulin A. *Gastroenterology*, **60**, 1.
47. Tomasi, T. B. (1972) Secretory immunoglobulins. *New. Eng. Med. J.*, **287**, 500.
48. Wright, R. N. and Rothberg, R. M. (1971) The reactions of pepsin and pepsin-trysin digestion products of bovine serum albumin with antisera from rabbits ingesting this protein. *J. Immunol.*, **107**, 1410.
49. Schwartz, D. P. and Buckley, R. H. (1971) Serum IgE concentrations and skin reactivity to anti IgE antibody in IgG deficient patients. *New. Eng. Med. J.*, **284**, 513.
50. Tada, T. and Ishizaka, K. (1970) Distribution of γE forming cells in lymphoid tissues of the human and monkey. *J. Immunol.*, **104**, 377.
51. Stanworth, D. R. (1970) Immunochemical mechanisms of immediate type hypersensitivity reactions. *Clin. exp. Immunol.*, **6**, 1.
52. Stanworth, D. R. (1971) The experimental inhibition of reagin mediated reactions. *Clin. Allergy*, **1**, 25.
53. Stevenson, D. D., Orgel, A. H., Hamburger, R. N., Reid, R. T. and Richardson, D. E. (1971) Development of IgE in newborn human infants. *J. Allergy appl. Immunol.*, **48**, 61.
54. Kaufman, H. S. (1971) Allergy in the newborn. Skin test reactions confirmed by the Prausnitz–Küstner test at birth. *Clin. Allergy*, **1**, 363.
55. Matthews, T. S. and Soothill, J. F. (1970) Complement activation after milk feeding in children with cow's milk allergy. *Lancet*, **II**, 893.
56. Freier, S. (1973) In: Clinical Immunology in Paediatric Medicine. Report of the First Unigate Paediatric Workshop. Ed. by Brostoff, J. Oxford: Blackwell Scientific.
57. Morris, D. L. (1969) Use of sublingual antigen in diagnosis and treatment of food allergy. *Annls Allergy*, **27**, 289.
58. Hoffman, D. R. and Haddad, Z. H. (1974) Diagnosis of IgE mediated reactions to

food antigens by radioimmunoassay. *J. Allergy Clin. Immunol.*, **54**, 3, 165.
59. Johansson, S. G. O., Bennich, H., Berg, T. and Foucard, T. (1973) The clinical significance of IgE antibody in serum as determined by RAST. In: *Mechanisms in Allergy Reagin—Mediated Hypersensitivity.* Ed. by Goodfriend, L., Sehon, A. H. and Orange, R. P. New York: Marcel Dekker.
60. Heiner, D. C. (1975) The use of RAST in the study of allergy to food. In: *Advances in Diagnosis of Allergy: RAST.* Ed. by Evans, R., p. 153. Miami: Medical Book Publishers.
61. Hoffman, D. R., Yamamoto, F. Y., Geller, B. D. and Haddad, Z. H. (1975) Specific IgE antibodies in atopic eczema. *J. Allergy Clin. Immunol.*, **55**, 526.
62. Hoffman, D. R. (1975) Food allergy in children: RAST studies with milk and egg. In: *Advances in Diagnosis of Allergy: RAST.* Ed. by Evans, R., p. 165. Miami: Medical Book Publishers.
63. Jarrett, E. E. (1977) Activation of IgE regulatory mechanisms by transmucosal absorption of antigen. *Lancet*, **II**, 223.
64. Rowe, A. H. (1944) *Elimination Diets and the Patient's Allergies. A Handbook of Allergy.* 2nd ed. Philadelphia: Lea and Febiger.
65. Sheldon, J. M., Mathews, K. P. and Lovell. R. B. (1967) *A Manual of Clinical Allergy.* 2nd ed. Philadelphia: Saunders.
66. Paulsen, H. C. (1961) Alimentary allergy. Allergy to fish. *Acta allerg.*, **16**, 380.
67. Francis, D. E. M. and Dixon, D. J. W. (1970) *Diets for Sick Children.* 2nd ed. Oxford: Blackwell Scientific.
68. Taylor, K. B., Truelove, S. C., Thomson, D. L. and Wright, R. (1961) An immunological study of coeliac disease and idiopathic steatorrhea: serological reactions to gluten and milk proteins. *Br. med. J.*, **II**, 1727.
69. Asquith, P., Thompson, R. A. and Cooke, W. T. (1969) Serum immunoglobulins in coeliac disease. *Lancet*, **II**, 129.
70. Perrett, A. D., Higgins, G., Johnston, H. H., Massarella, G. R., Truelove, S. C. and Wright, R. (1971) The liver in Crohn's disease. *Q. J. Med.*, **40**, 187.
71. Gelzayd, E. A., Kraft, S. C., Fitch, F. W. and Kirsner, J. B. (1968) Distribution of immunoglobulins in human rectal mucosa. Ulcerative colitis and abnormal mucosal control subjects. *Gastroenterology*, **54**, 341.
72. Collins-Williams, C. (1955) Acute allergic reactions to cow's milk. *Annls Allergy*, **13**, 415.
73. Ament, M. E. and Rubin, C. E. (1972) Soy protein—another cause of the flat intestinal lesion. *Gastroenterology*, **61**, 227.
74. Mendoza, J. and Meyers, J. (1970) Soybean sensitivity: Case report. *Pediatrics*, **46**, 774.
75. Halpin, T. C., Byrne, W. J. and Ament, M. E. (1977) Colitis, persistent diarrhoea and soy protein intolerance. *J. Pediatr.*, **91**, 404.
76. Visakorpi, J. P. and Immonen, P. (1967) Intolerance to cow's milk and wheat gluten in the primary malabsorption syndrome in infancy. *Acta paediatr. Scand.*, **56**, 49.
77. Bleumink, E. and Young, E. (1968) Identification of the atopic allergen in cow's milk. *Int. archs. Allergy appl. Immunol.*, **37**, 5.
78. Freier, S. and Berger, H. (1973) Disodium cromoglycate in gastrointestinal protein intolerance. *Lancet*, **II**, 916.
79. Shiner, M., Ballard, J. and Smith, M. E. (1975) The small intestinal mucosa in cow's milk allergy. *Lancet*, **I**, 136.
80. Hall, J. G., Levin, J., Kuhn, J., Ottenheimer, E., Van Berkum, P. and McKusick, V. A. (1969) Thrombocytopoenia with absent radius (TAR). *Medicine*, **48**, 411.
81. Whitfield, M. F. and Barr, D. G. D. (1976) Cow's milk allergy in the syndrome of thrombocytopoenia with absent radius. *Arch. Dis. Child.*, **51**, 337.
82. McNeish, A. S. (1974) The role of lactose in cow's milk intolerance. *Acta Paediatrica Scand.*, **63**, 652.
83. Kuitunen, P., Visakorpi, J. P., Savilathi, E. and Pelkonen, P. (1975) Malabsorption syndrome with cow's milk intolerance: Clinical findings and course in 54 cases. *Archs. dis. Child.*, **50**, 351.

84. Kuitunen, P., Rapola, J., Savilathi, E., Visakorpi, J. P. (1973) Response of the jejunal mucosa to cow's milk in the malabsorption syndrome with cow's milk intolerance; a light and electron microscope study. *Acta paediatr. Scand.*, **62**, 585.

85. Fontaine, J. L. and Navarro, J. (1975) Small intestinal biopsy in cow's milk protein allergy in infancy. *Archs. dis. Child.*, **50**, 357.

86. Kuzemko, J. A. and Simpson, K. R. (1977) Unpublished data.

87. Kilby, A., Walker-Smith, J. A. and Wood, C. B. S. (1975) Small intestinal mucosa in cow's milk allergy. *Lancet*, **I**, 531.

88. Harrison, M., Kilby, A., Walker-Smith, J. A., France, N. E. and Wood, C. B. S. (1976) Cow's milk protein intolerance: A possible association with gastroenteritis, lactose intolerance and IgA deficiency. *Br. med. J.*, **1**, 1501.

89. Kuzemko, J. A. and Simpson, K. R. (1974) Treatment of allergy to cow's milk. *Lancet*, **I**, 338.

90. Freier, S. (1977) A therapeutic trial of disodium cromoglycate in gastrointestinal allergy. *Allergolog. Immunopathol.*, **5**, 450.

91. Mani, V., Lloyd, G., Green, F. H. Y., Fox, H. and Turberg, L. A. (1976) Treatment of ulcerative colitis with oral disodium cromoglycate. *Lancet*, **I**, 439.

92. Heatley, E. V., Calcroft, B. J., Rhodes, J., Owen, E. and Evans, B. K. (1975) Disodium cromoglycate in the treatment of chronic proctitis. *Gut*, **16**, 559.

93. Chu, J., O'Connor, D. M., McElfesh, A. D. and Mueller, J. (1976) *Gastritis varioliformis*, allergy and disodium cormoglycate. *Lancet*, **I**, 964.

94. Dolovich, J., Punthakee, N. D., MacMillan, A. B. and Osbaldeston, G. J. (1974) Systemic mastocytosis: Control of diarrhoea by ingested disodium cromoglycate. *Can. med. Ass. J.*, **III**, 684.

95. Bock, S. A., Buckley, J., Holst, A. and May, C. D. (1977) Proper use of skin tests with food extracts in diagnosis of hypersensitivity to food in children. *Clin. Allergy*, **7**, 375.

96. Scheinmann, P., Gendrel, J., Charlas, J. and Paupe, J. (1976) Value of lymphoblast transformation test in cow's milk protein intestinal intolerance. *Clin. Allergy*, **6**, 515.

97. Dannaeus, T., Fouchard, T. and Johansson, S. G. O. (1977) The effect of orally administered sodium cromoglycate on symptoms of food allergy. *Clin. Allergy*, **7**, 109.

98. Russell, F. and Shaw, M. D. (1975) Cromolyntherapy in chronic infantile eczema. *Arch Dermatol.*, **III**, 1537.

99. Galant, S. P., Bullock, J. and Frick, O. L. (1973) An immunological approach to the diagnosis of food sensitivity. *Clin. Allergy*, **3**, 363.

100. Walker, S. R., Evans, M. E., Richards, A. J. and Paterson, J. W. (1972) The fate of ^{14}C disodium cromoglycate in man. *J. Pharmacol.*, **24**, 525.

101. Kingsby, P. J. (1974) Oral sodium cromoglycate in gastrointestinal allergy. *Lancet*, **I**, 1011.

102. Westall, R. C. (1974) Dietary treatment of a child with maple syrup urine disease. (branched-chain ketoaciduria) *Archs. dis. Child.*, **38**, 485.

103. Beigler, M. A. (1971) The elemental diet: A new concept in nutritional support of the debilitated patient. *Surg. Digest*, **6**, 18.

104. Belin, R. P. (1970) Use of vivonex-100 in paediatric surgery. *Internal Symposium on Balanced Nutrition and Therapy*. Nuremberg.

105. Hyman, C. J., Reiter, J. and Rodnan, J. (1971) Parenteral and oral alimentation in the treatment of the non-specific protracted diarrhoeal syndrome of infancy. *J. Pediatr.*, **78**, 17.

106. Davidson, G. P., Hill, D. J. and Townley, R. R. W. (1976) Gastrointestinal milk allergy in childhood: A rational approach. *Med. J. Austral.*, 945.

107. Sumithran, E. and Iyngkaran, N. (1977) Is jejunal biopsy really necessary in cow's milk protein intolerance? *Lancet*, **I**, 1122.

108. Buissert, P. D. (1978) Common manifestations of cow's milk allergy in children. *Lancet*, **I**, 304.

109. Aas, K. (1978) The diagnosis of hypersensitivity to ingested foods. Reliability of skin prick testing and the radioallergosorbent test with different materials. *Clin. Allergy*, **8**, 39.

CHAPTER 5

Skin Allergy

IN MANAGING CHILDREN with a chronic skin condition, it is useful to remember that the child and his family are aware of and can follow its natural history because they can actually see it. For this simple reason one should always be sympathetic and take seriously any rash about which the mother has expressed concern. It is also worth stressing that many parents fear that their child's skin condition may be infectious and often forbid him to take part in various school and sporting activities, e.g. swimming. Such a course of action may cause emotional problems in the child.

One should, therefore, take time and explain in simple language the basic facts, the principles of management, and the outlook and stress that however unsightly the skin may appear, it will eventually heal completely without scarring. Time, patience and teaching the parents and the child how to cope with a chronic skin disease is not only a challenge to the doctor's skills, but also quite rewarding to his small patient.

Atopic dermatitis (atopic eczema—to break out, to boil over)

This is a chronic recurring disease of young children of uncertain aetiology although hereditary and allergic factors may be of great significance. As a rule the lesions are symmetrical and bilateral, and may occur anywhere on the body. In the young child, three phases are seen, all of which are associated with pruritus. Initially there is an erythema of the skin which proceeds to the formation of microvesicles (weeping). The result of such injury to the skin results in an increased epidermal activity and leads to scaling. In older children pigmentary changes are often observed, also a thickening of the skin.

The pathophysiological features demonstrate a vasodilatation which is accompanied by the release of various vasoactive substances such as histamine, kinins, serotonin, prostaglandins, acetycholine, etc. and invasion of the epidermis by inflammatory cells. The oedema which arises is responsible for the microvesicle formation and changes in the epidermis. The stratum corneum which is thus formed is imperfect and may show cells containing nuclei (parakeratosis). The thickening of the dermis and epidermis is due to the downward proliferation of the rete ridges (acanthosis).[1–5,10]

It is worth pointing out that this type of lesion can be seen in other dermatoses although there are exceptions, e.g. histiocytosis X.

The common skin conditions which will be discussed are shown in Table 5.1.

Table 5.1

Atopic dermatitis (atopic eczema)	Seborrheic dermatitis
Contact dermatitis	Infective dermatitis
Urticaria	Irritant dermatitis
	Nummular 'eczema'

Incidence and heredity

In about 80 per cent of infants a positive history of atopy is obtained.[1] If one or both parents suffer from atopic eczema the outlook for the child's dermatitis clearing up during childhood is poor.[12] The incidence of atopic eczema in children is between 3 and 5 per cent.[6–8] In an interesting study of identical twins, it was demonstrated that although both twins developed atopic eczema during childhood, it did not occur simultaneously.[14,15] About 60 per cent of children with atopic eczema eventually develop asthma, allergic rhinitis or some other atopic disease.[8,11–13] About 10 per cent of children with atopic dermatitis have ichthyosis which will persist once atopic eczema has cleared. It is also of interest that adolescents with acne and those who have a family history of acne have a reduced incidence of atopic dermatitis.[9] It is suggestive that atopic dermatitis in young children is more common in the well developed industrialised nations of the world that in the rural ones. For instance, children of West Indian families who have moved to England have an increased incidence compared to children in Jamaica.[17] Similar findings were observed in Chinese children in the United States.[18]

Few studies have been published on the natural history of eczema. In one study 50 per cent of individuals still had atopic eczema at the age of 20 and half of them also had asthma.[11] In a study of 218 children who were reviewed 10 years after the initial diagnosis, it was found that in 17 per cent there was no change in the clinical state of atopic eczema, 13 per cent had minor flexural lesions, and 70 per cent normal skins. In general, in about 75 to 80 per cent of children atopic eczema develops during the first year of life. In the majority it will subside by the third birthday and may temporarily recur (for weeks or months) at 5 to 7 years and around puberty. Children who have symptoms beyond their third birthday will usually show some skin features as adults. In a minority of children atopic eczema will start during late childhood.[16]

Immunological aspects

The majority of children with atopic dermatitis over a period of time develop high serum IgE levels, although little correlation exists between the severity of the condition and the degree of elevation of IgE. Some studies have shown that the level of IgE has a tendency to fluctuate with the clinical condition. In many children the level of IgE returns to normal when atopic eczema clears up spontaneously.[19-21] Such normal levels may also be shown in children who have patches of flexural atopic eczema or in those with nummular eczema.[20,30] However, it is not accepted by some authorities that atopic eczema is caused by IgE mediated allergy. They feel that antigen—antibody reactions are responsible for exacerbations of the condition because the skin is abnormal and because atopic dermatitis can develop in children who have no IgE at all.[49] It is well known that such children have hyper-active skins which differ in responses to various physical and pharmacological agents, e.g. white dermographism, abnormal responses to temperature changes and paradoxical responses to histamine and acetycholine (delayed blanch phenomenon).[13,23,24] Children with atopic dermatitis show very weak skin sensitivity responses to antigens or even anaphylactic reactions, e.g. human dander.[25] Recent studies suggest that leucocytes may show chemotactic abnormalities although such reduced chemotaxis was not related to the severity of atopic eczema, the serum IgE levels, or an infection. Nevertheless phagocytes not only destroy bacteria but handle the antigen at the site of penetration, hence defect in phagocytic function may well be of critical importance.[110-112] It would seem, therefore, that just as the bronchi of an asthmatic child show increased hyper-reactivity similar features may occur in the skin.

Skin blood vessels of children with atopic eczema also show abnormal responses. For instance, pronounced vasoconstriction occurs on exposure to cold. This feature is thought to be related to the release of acetycholine because intradermal injection of mecholyl causes blanching in at least 70 per cent of all individuals with atopic eczema.[24,26,27,29] This observation has been documented in the new born baby, but whether it can be used as a predictive test of atopy remains uncertain because apparently normal subjects may show similar responses.[28] Although sweating may aggravate atopic eczema, it is not known whether any allergens are actually excreted in the sweat thus exerting a deleterious effect on the condition. The dry skin is thought to be due to the reduced sebaceous gland activity, decrease in fat content and sweat retention.[2,10,31] In an interesting study[32] it was found that babies treated with diets containing a reduction in calories and no linoleic acid developed dry skin and eczema in the intertriginous areas. The condition cleared up after treatment with linoleic acid. Similar observations can be seen in patients maintained for a long time on intravenous feeding.[33,34]

Areas of the body covered by the atopic dermatitis appear to itch excessively and over-react to any minor stimulus which may be due to enhanced skin sensitivity. Scratching, lichenification (thickening of the epidermis), superficial and often spreading infection occurs, leading in turn to more scratching and thus deterioration of the skin condition. Although subjects with atopic eczema scratch often during sleep, the bouts of scratching last considerably longer when the individual is awake than during sleep states.[35-37]

Clinical features

The age of onset of atopic eczema is, as a rule, after the first 4 weeks of life and by the age of 3 years about 80 per cent of eczematous children would have developed the condition. In the baby it starts on the face, ears and scalp. It is uncommon to see atopic eczema over the napkin area. By the age of 2 years exposed surfaces of the body such as extensor aspects of the knees, ankles and elbows are affected. The lesions show weeping, vesicle formation and scaling. There is a fair amount of itching. In older children the lesions proceed to lichenification (thickening). Over the years there is a tendency to spontaneous improvement although many children have exacerbations during puberty. Children whose atopic eczema becomes infected may have enlarged regional lymph nodes, which disappear following effective treatment.

The relationship of seborrhoeic dermatitis, dermatitis of the scalp (cradle cap) to atopic eczema remains uncertain. It is true that some babies with seborrheic dermatitis or cradle cap eventually develop typical lesions of atopic dermatitis. There is indeed enormous similarity between these lesions and atopic eczema. Cradle cap is possibly a variant of seborrhoeic dermatitis; it disappears in most babies by the third or fourth week of life. However, in some children the dermatitis persists and spreads down, involving ears, forehead, and flexural regions of elbows and knees. There is little itching. After a few weeks the eruption has a tendency to heal spontaneously but in a minority of infants it evolves into typical lesions of atopic dermatitis.

Although children with atopic eczema are not more prone to develop allergic contact dermatitis than normal children, they may sometimes tolerate contactants poorly, e.g. wool, lanolin. Children with eczema should not be vaccinated against smallpox as the risk of vaccinia is great

and such children are particularly liable to develop severe infections with
Herpes simplex virus. Adolescents who have had atopic eczema for many
years may develop keratoconus (conical cornea) and cataracts.
Keratoconus is a degenerative change in the cornea which interferes with
vision and can be satisfactorily treated by wearing contact lenses. Atopic
cataracts are bilateral, and may appear over a period of years, but occasionally may arise within 2 or 3 weeks and at the time when there is a
flare-up of eczema.

During the first few weeks of life atopic dermatitis should be distinguished from infective and irritant dermatitis. Infective dermatitis has
a tendency to involve napkin areas and occasionally the face. The lesions
are weeping and there is much crusting. Occasionally skin ulcers are seen
especially on the buttocks. There is very little itching and when the condition has been present for some time satellite lesions spread to other
parts of the body. Skin cultures are usually positive for *Candida
albicans, Staphylococcus aureus,* streptococci or some other pathogen.

Irritant dermatitis occurs within the first month of life and involves
particularly the napkin area. Lesions are red and weeping. There is very
little scaling and itching. Satellite lesions are rarely seen unless there is a
secondary infection. Skin cultures are as a rule negative.

Other conditions which may be confused with atopic eczema in the
young child include Ritter's disease (toxic epidermal necrolysis, scalded
skin syndrome) due to infection with phage type 71 or 55/71
Staphylococcus aureus, contact dermatitis, insect bites, over-exposure of
the baby to extremes of temperature and congenital ichthyosiform
erythroderma (skin rash from birth, electron microscopic examination of
skin diagnostic).

It is important to remember that atopic eczema-like lesions may be
present or be the presenting feature in a group of important systematic
diseases of children. Some of these are ennumerated in Table 5.2.

Nummular 'eczema' is a term given to round aggregations of papules
and vesicles which may occur in the atopic or non-atopic child (num-
mulus—coin). The lesions, which cause itching, measure about 1–5 cm
diameter and are predominantly found on the hands and feet but may be
more widespread. Serum IgE levels are normal.[64] The natural history and
management is similar to atopic dermatitis.

Diagnosis

The diagnosis of atopic dermatitis is straightforward and can be sup-
ported by a number of laboratory investigations.

Allergy skin testing. Skin prick tests to various foods, especially egg

Table 5.2

Condition	Remarks
Immune deficiency states:	
Leiner's d	Dermatitis within the first few days of life becoming generalised. Diarrhoea and a tendency to infection. Defect in function of fifth component of complement (C_5). May be familial[38-40]
Wiskott–Aldrich S	Dermatitis within first few days of life. Thrombocytopenia and infections. Low serum IgM. Recessive[41,42,50,51]
Ataxia–telangiectasia	Dermatitis occurs in 10%. Low serum IgA[43,46]
Agammaglobulinanaemia (sex-linked)	Dermatitis occurs in 5%. Low serum IgA and IgG[43,49]
Chronic granulomatous D (Job's S)	Sex linked or autosmal recessive. Generalised 'cold' staphylococcal infections[44,45,53]
Hereditary skin diseases:	
Acrokeratotic poikiloderma (Rothmund–Thomson S)	Photosensitive dermatitis. Sparse hair and eye lashes. Skin telangiectases[47]
Anhidrotic ectodermal dysplasia	Flexural areas affected. May have asthma and/or allergic rhinitis[48]
Ichtyosis and other features[52,58] a. Cockayne S	Photosensitive dermatitis, small stature, enlarged liver and spleen, bone and eye abnormalities
b. Netherton S	Generalised dermatitis, asthma and/or allergic rhinitis may be present. Scalp hair fragile (bamboo hair). Aminoaciduria.
c. Sjögren–Larson S	Dermatitis and neurological involvement
Metabolic diseases:	
Phenylketonuria	Dermatitis ten times greater than in general population[54]
Hartnup's d	Photosensitive dermatitis of exposed parts of the body[54]
Ahistidinaemia	Generalised dermatitis in children on low histidine diet[55]
Mucopolysaccharidoses	Dermatitis seen occasionally. Skin is generally thickened but isolated nodules may be felt[49]

Table 5.2 (*continued*)

Condition	Remarks
Chromosome anomalies:	
Deletion of Long arm 18	Generalised dermatitis, microcephaly, small stature and skeletal abnormalities[56,57]
Miscellaneous conditions:	
Histiocytosis X	Dermatitis a feature of Letterer–Siwe's d. Hands, neck and napkin areas involved[52]
Acrodermatitis enteropathica	Dermatitis often the presenting feature. Involves buccal, napkin areas and exposed arms. Nail involvement present[59,60]
Gluten-induced enteropathy	Dermatitis occasionally seen usually involving face and hands[61]
Bloom's S	Photosensitive dermatitis, low birth weight, malar hypoplasia, small stature[62]
Dubowitz's S	Generalised dermatitis, small stature, ptosis, shallow supra-orbital ridges[63]

white, are positive in at least 80 per cent of children under the age of 2 years. However, if such positive skin tests are followed by challenges with specific foods, no change in atopic eczema is observed. In some children anaphylactic reactions can be seen such as vomiting or urticaria. Skin tests are rarely necessary to confirm the diagnosis of atopic eczema but they may be useful in a child who has already developed other features of allergy such as rhinitis or asthma.

IgE. As has been mentioned before, exceedingly high concentrations of serum IgE are found in children with atopic dermatitis, and there is a tendency for such levels to persist for many months after the condition has settled down.

Blood eosinophilia. A total eosinophil count is often raised and may correlate well with the severity of the clinical features.

Treatment

It is important during the first interview to discuss with the mother the natural history of the condition, its complications, contra-indications to immunisation and long term management. The following general remarks should be made:

Hygiene. Drying soaps should be avoided. Fatted soaps and shampoos are best, e.g. any baby soap. Nails should be kept short to reduce the damage from scratching.

Weather conditions. Children with atopic eczema dislike a hot and humid atmosphere because it makes them perspire excessively resulting in irritation and pruritus. The parents should be advised against over-dressing their child and be guided by daily weather conditions. The skin irritation and itching often leads to scratching and thus secondary bacterial infection. Indeed, it has been shown that such lesions and surrounding areas are often major foci of pathogenic staphylococci[65]—a feature which is not observed in some other skin conditions, e.g. psoriasis. Scratching may occur during the child's sleep but mostly it is a problem throughout the day. Hence, parents should be advised to keep the living room and bedroom temperatures fairly even at around 18–20°C, to use cotton sheets, light synthetic blankets or a duvet. At all times extremes of temperatures should be avoided.

Clothing. Cotton and soft synthetic materials are well tolerated. Other materials tend to irritate the skin especially woollen clothes and plastic napkins.

Diet. The reasons for trying an elimination diet should be discussed and it should be pointed out that occasionally a diet may be successful if used in a baby of 6 months of age or under. Some parents may wish to try the effect of goat's milk. They should be encouraged as from time to time atopic eczema does clear during the duration of goat's milk treatment.

This may be a good time to discuss breast feeding and encourage the mother, without making her feel guilty, to breast feed any future babies. However, the doctor should decide for himself when is the most opportune moment to discuss the subject of breast feeding.

Bathing. There exists a fair amount of controversy regarding the benefits of bathing in children with atopic dermatitis. There are those who forbid it at all times,[97] and others who recommend frequent or twice weekly baths. It is argued that children with atopic eczema have dry skins, hence, frequent bathing will lead to more dryness unless artificial barriers are applied by using oily applications. The simplest and the most effective way to do this is by using an emulsifying ointment B.P. which is added to the bath water. The mother should dissolve one or two tablespoonfuls of the ointment in a litre of boiling water and mix it with the bath water. The water should be tepid as very hot water can cause skin irritation. Once the child is in the water, all parts of his body should be gently massaged and if any of the other sibling wish to join such activity he should be encouraged. During the initial acute stage of atopic dermatitis such baths can be given daily and gradually reduced as healing occurs. At all times they should be used at least once weekly. It is not necessary and may indeed be harmful to add antiseptic solutions to the bath. Emulsifying ointment baths are useful in children with severe and generalised skin conditions but are unnecessary when small areas of the body are affected. Other approaches, such as the modified Scholtz regimen,[73] i.e. use of non-cleansing lotion, containing cetaphil (a non-lipid) has its protagonists, mostly in North America.[72]

School activities and play. The child should be encouraged to lead as normal a life as possible and to partake in all school games and activities. If a child is keen on swimming, it should be pointed out that chlorinated water may act as an irritant but if he is keen on such an activity, he should be strongly encouraged. If desired a barrier cream can be applied to the skin before swimming or in more widely spread eczema, he should take a bath with an emulsifying ointment once he returns home. Swimming in the sea as a rule does not present any problems as salty water is helpful. Indeed, sea air (low humidity, dust free, cool, high intensity ultraviolet light) is often very beneficial.

Immunisations and vaccinations. As mentioned earlier a child with atopic dermatitis is particularly prone to develop *Herpes simplex* infections (eczema herpetiformis), and vaccinial infections (kaposi varicelliform eruption or eczema vaccinatum). Similar lesions can be produced by other viruses,[66,67] e.g. the Coxsackie viruses. Vaccination, therefore, against smallpox is absolutely contra-indicated and contact with other siblings or individuals who have been recently vaccinated should be strongly avoided. Rarely because of the presence of smallpox in a locality, or because of travel to an endemic area, primary vaccination of children with eczema can be employed using an attenuated vaccinia virus. In all such children vaccinia immunoglobulin (0·4 mg/kg i.m.) should be given at the same time. The management of eczema vaccinatum, which carries about 5 per cent mortality, includes the use of methisazone and immunoglobulin.[68-70] Other immunisations are well tolerated but precautions should be taken in children with egg sensitivity as some vaccines are made on embryonated hens' eggs.

Psychological factors. In general, psychological factors are uncommon in children with atopic eczema, and they tend to be mild in nature, and are secondary to the complications of the condition, e.g. intense itching. Nevertheless, the effect of psyche on skin should be fully discussed and simple advice offered.

Hyposensitisation. No objective evidence exists in the literature that hyposensitisation is of benefit in children with atopic dermatitis. One placebo-control study showed that if the child's eczema could be proven to be associated with a specific inhalant allergen, immunotherapy might be useful.[71] We have not found hyposensitisation of value and because of the complications would not recommend its routine use in children under the age of 7 years.

Local applications. No evidence exists that any local skin treatment influences the prognosis of atopic dermatitis. Undoubtedly the many skin preparations currently used in treatment shorten exacerbations but they may also lead to undesirable side-effects.

Topical corticosteroids. The beneficial effects of topical steroids in atopic dermatitis are obtained by virtue of their anti-inflammatory, immunosuppressive and vasoconstrictive actions. However, acute tolerance (tachyphylaxis or rapid diminution of a pharmacological response with repeated uses of the drug) rapidly develops, and is especially prominent with fluorinated corticosteroids. Thus, for instance, after 30 to 50 hours, one dose of a topical steroid is as effective as three or five applications. The mechanism of tachyphylaxis remains uncertain but may involve the production of skin catecholamines. In addition steroids have been shown to remain in the stratum corneum for as long as 30 days, and some, such as the fluorinated agents, appear to be absorbed systemically quite easily. Administration of topical steroids in conditions associated with skin infections, especially fungal or viral, is contra-indicated. Not only do they inhibit the weal defence mechanisms but may also significantly alter the natural progression of the disease and confuse the clinical picture.[13,49,74-79]

Prolonged systemic absorption of topical corticosteroids may lead to suppression of the hypothalmic–pituitary–adrenal axis and growth failure. Local side-effects include thinning of the skin, striae especially in flexural areas, telangiectasia and occasionally bruising (most often seen on the face).[75,80-82]

It is important to remember that a child who has a dry skin will often do better when ointment is used (no water) whereas a child who has weepy, moist skin will prefer cream as it causes less irritation than ointments which remain on the skin for a long time. Moreover, some ointments and creams contain additives, e.g. lanolin, preservative agents, etc. which may in themselves lead to skin irritation. It is important therefore, to check the contents of the preparation most carefully.

The huge number of topical corticosteroid preparations with differing pack sizes and differing dosage dilutions have been a hindrance rather than a help in the management of atopic dermatitis. Short lived successes with the most potent and recently introduced preparations are usually widely reported leading to unnecessary confusion. Moreover, some doctors use these agents empirically and since it is virtually impossible to be certain as to the actual amounts of an application used daily or weekly, different views and approaches are expressed regarding treatment.

The following therefore, is the scheme we use and which we offer as a guideline.

a. 0·5 or 1 per cent hydrocortisone twice daily is applied for full 3 days or until such time as skin healing occurs. Subsequent treatments are given intermittently at the time of any flare up and for a maximum of 3 days.

b. If it is suspected that secondary bacterial infection might be present, swabs are taken and systemic erythromycin given four times daily for 7 days. We find such an approach superior to topical administration of antibiotics, or steroid–antibiotic combinations.

c. Daily or twice weekly bath with emulsifying oil B.P. are continued throughout.

d. The child's condition is reviewed every 1, 2 or 3 weeks and aspects of general management discussed.

e. If at any time there is *severe* exacerbation of the dermatitis, Betnovate (1:5 dilution) in liquid and soft yellow paraffin is used once daily after a bath for up to 7 days and strict instruction issued that it should never be applied on the face as inadvertent application to the eyes may cause damage. We believe that the very potent topical corticosteroids such as clobetasol proprionate 0·05 per cent, fluocinonide 0·05 per cent, desonite 0·05 per cent etc. have little additional value in young children.

f. If it is suspected that the mother might have applied more than 25 g of a steroid within 1 month, a synacthen test of adrenal function is performed and repeated periodically.[83]

g. Topical corticosteroids are often of little value in the older child with nummular eczema. Such children often obtain benefit from Lassar's paste which contains 1 per cent crude coal tar. Although there are many refined preparations of tar, undoubtedly the crude tar is the most effective. Preferably tar preparations should be applied during the winter and autumn months as the tar itself may sensitise the skin to sunlight and cause an intense reaction.

h. During the initial stages of eczema when the child has intense itching and irritation, it is beneficial to prescribe an evening dose of an antihistamine such as trimeprazine tartrate (0·5 mg/kg) which appears to be particularly effective. We have not found any other agents or drugs of superior value.

i. If an ichthyotic child develops severe generalised eczema, it is worth considering ultraviolet light treatment. However, before such course of action is taken, one should carefully discuss the object of treatment and management with the parents as some children's eczema deteriorates following ultraviolet light exposure.

j. The use of non-steroid preparations and 10 per cent sodium cromoglycate ointment in the management of children with atopic dermatitis is currently being investigated. Early results are promising.[96]

Contact dermatitis

Contact dermatitis is of two types:

    a. Primary irritant contact dermatitis.
    b. Allergic contact dermatitis.

Primary irritant dermatitis is caused by substances which are in contact with the skin for prolonged periods and cause epidermal damage. The most common irritants are organic solvents, detergents, and alkalis. Temperature may also exert an irritant effect.

Allergic contact dermatitis is caused by the binding of proteins in the epidermis with exogenous chemical agents forming complete antigens. The reaction which occurs is mediated by the delayed or Type IV (Coombs and Gell) classification mechanism. An immediate or Type I reaction is often triggered off in the process.[84,85] The inflammatory changes which result are caused by various chemical mediators such as histamine, acetylcholine, prostaglandins of the E and F series, slow reacting substance-A (SRS-A) and possible other agents. The involvement of cyclic AMP in the release of such mediators remains unclear.[5,86,87]

Although histological features of allergic contact dermatitis and primary irritant dermatitis are very similar, fine distinguishing features can be observed on electron microscopy such as lysosomes and spongiosis.[88]

Clinical features

Well defined patches of skin show redness, weeping, vesicle or bullous formation, swelling, scaling and thickening of the skin. Itching is always present.

Contact dermatitis occurs in older children and adolescents. Family history or personal history of atopy is absent.

The lesions commonly affect hands, face, eyelids, neck, legs and occasionally the perianal area. The surrounding skin is normal. A simple guide illustrating the parts of the body affected and possible aetiological agents is shown in Table 5.3.

Table 5.3

Part of body	Possible aetological agent
Scalp	Lotions, shampoos
Eyelids	Creams, dyes
Face	Cosmetics (from mother's hands and face)
Ears	Nickel sulphate, metal frames
Nose	Nasal drops, paper tissues
Lips and perioral region	Lipstick
Neck	Cosmetics, dyes, metal, scarves
Axillae	Deodorants
Hands and forearms	Gloves, soap, plants
Trunk	Clothing
Thighs and legs	Clothing, under-garments
Feet	Shoes, dyes, tanning agents

Potential sensitisers

The number of chemicals to which an individual can be exposed in every day life is almost limitless. For instance, a perfume can contain at least a thousand substances. It is not surprising, therefore, that young children can be sensitised to chemicals during the first few years of life. Common sensitisers are various topical medications which may include antibiotics, anaesthetic agents, antihistamines, ethylinediamine, paraben mixtures, dyes, metals, cosmetics, etc.

Young girls may develop nickel sulphate dermatitis if they have had their ears pierced. Initially such dermatitis is observed around the ear lobes and subsequently round the neck from a necklace or some other article or garment containing nickel sulphate.

Diagnosis and investigation

A careful and detailed history will establish the cause in the majority of children and can be confirmed by patch testing. Total serum IgE and eosinophil counts are within normal limits. A number of *in vitro* tests have been devised to establish definitive diagnosis and these include the migration inhibition test,[90] the lymphocyte transformation test,[89,91] and the application of the patch testing technique in certain animals.[84] None of these investigations has so far established itself as a useful and reproducible tool in routine clinical work.

Patch test. Fabre[92] observed skin blisters caused by caterpillars and demonstrated a test technique which is basically the same as is used today in clinical medicine. The suspected substance is applied to an area of normal skin for 48–72 hours and is held in place by an adhesive tape.

After this time the skin is inspected and examined for erythema, papules and vesicles.

Systemic corticosteroids and other drugs should be avoided during patch testing because they modify the response.[93]

Method. Use the back provided the skin is healthy and not affected by an episode of dermatitis. (The back is more sensitive than the arms.)

Use allergens which are pure and of known concentration.

Use a control patch.

If liquid—place a few drops on 2 cm square piece of filter paper, cover with 2·5 cm square piece of polythene film and seal with an adhesive tape so as to occlude completely all borders.

A convenient strip of test patches made from cellulose paper with polythene films and aluminium foils is commercially available (A1-test, Imeco, Sweden).

Apply disc to skin and seal with adhesive tape. Remove the patch test after 48 hr—record findings. Review the skin after a further 48 hr. (About 10 per cent of subjects will show reaction on second inspection only.)

Ask the mother to observe the patch area daily for 7 days and notify you of any reactions.

Positive reactions can be recorded as follows:

Erythema	+
Erythema, swelling, papules	+++
Erythema, swelling, papules, vesicles	++++
Blisters	+++++

At all times beware of toxic reactions. If uncertain repeat the test again, or use different dilutions. Complications are rarely encountered but may include exacerbation of dermatitis, necrosis, secondary infection, systemic absorption causing effects in other parts of the body or active sensitisation.[94] A list of concentrations for test substances can be obtained from published data.[95] In general 0·1 per cent solutions are the best to start with and concentrations can be increased gradually depending on clinical findings.

Treatment

Elimination of the cause. In the majority of instances no other therapy is required. During an acute severe episode a course of oral corticosteroids should be given, e.g. prednisolone for 3–5 days. Topical steroids are of no value in such cases, but may bring relief in the very mild exacerbation or mild chronic situations, e.g. erythema only. 1 per cent hydrocortisone ointment is a very satisfactory preparation. Hyposensitisation is of no beneficial value in any type of contact dermatitis.

Photo contact dermatitis

Very occasionally a child who has been using antiseptic soap may develop contact dermatitis following exposure to sunlight. A patch test site exposed to light for 12 hours will usually be positive.[98]

Urticaria (from *Urtica urens* or nettle plant)

Urticaria may be defined as a transient eruption of weals or circumscribed swellings in the skin often associated with pruritus and lasting for a few minutes, or few hours, but rarely over 48 hours. Acute urticaria is very common in childhood. The chronic recurrent form is very much less so. Angioedema (dry urticaria) is a term used when the condition involves the subcutaneous tissues.

Some of the common causes of urticaria in children are shown in Table 5.4.

Table 5.4

Causes of urticaria	Examples
Infections	Bacteria (local or general)
	Virus esp. Coxackie A9
	Fungus
	esp. due to trichophytan
Parasites	Ascariasis or oxyuriasis
Drugs	Almost any, esp. aspirin, penicillin.
Foods	Cow's milk, food additives
Contactants	Soaps, cosmetics, powders, detergents
Inhalants	Sprays, animal dander, feathers
Insect bites	Esp. flea bites
Psychogenic	
Physical agents	Sun, heat and cold, exercise
Associated with systemic diseases	Hodgkin's D
	Stevens–Johnson S., ulcerative colitis, etc.

Incidence

As has been pointed out earlier, the overall incidence of urticaria is not truly known because of the transient nature of the condition. The reported incidence varies between 0·5 and 16 per cent of the population.[99,100–102] For instance, in an English study of 3500 families the incidence of urticaria was 5·7 per cent.[103] In general about 3 per cent of children develop urticaria.[104] In a 12 year study of 554 patients referred to hospital with urticaria and angioedema, in 438 subjects no definite cause was evident; in 17 urticaria was associated with allergy; and in 19 was due to physical causes; in 28 it was associated with responses mediated by cholinergic sympathetic fibres; 47 with mechanical stimulation of the skin; 3 with pregnancy and 2 associated with the hereditary angioedema.[105] Both acute and chronic forms of urticaria are slightly more common in the females.[105,106]

Although allergy is not a common cause of urticaria the child who gives a past history of atopic eczema, asthma or pollenosis has considerably higher incidence of acute and chronic urticaria than a child with negative history of atopy.[106] In the majority of instances, the allergy causing urticaria is easily identified and clinical features appear to be mild and of shorter duration.

Pathogenesis

Urticaria results from localised vasodilation and transudation of fluid. Such a skin reaction may be produced by different stimuli, e.g. by pharmacological mediators which may be themselves abnormal, or by external agents or immunological factors. Thus, weal formation can result from the action of mediators of Type 1 reaction, as a manifestation of generalised anaphylaxis, or from Type II and Type III hypersensitivity reactions.[107]

Immunological aspects

Urticaria associated with allergic reactions has been fully studied and it is possible that allergy is responsible for the many so far unidentified instances of urticaria. The majority of acute allergic urticarial episodes are due to Type I hypersensitivity reactions. The total levels of IgE may be raised in acute urticaria but are normal in chronic states.[108] Some children with chronic urticaria and non-specific infections may have depressed serum levels of IgA, IgG and IgM.[109] Type I reactions may be responsible for those children who have food protein sensitivity, and may occur in association with certain drugs. Reactions to drugs however can be mediated by Type III reactions and also by various pharmacological mechanisms, some of which have been fully studied and some which remain still unknown. Type II reactions may occur in response to a byproduct of complement activation, but so far there exists little evidence that cytotoxic reactions are responsible for urticarial states. Type III reactions are fairly common, for instance as a part of serum sickness complex and following hyposensitising injections. The antigens commonly involved are foreign proteins and drugs. It is often possible to measure circulating IgG precipitating type antibody or IgG within urticarial lesions.[113] Although Type IV reactions may be involved in atopic eczema, and although other cutaneous vascular reactions have been described due to the release of prostaglandins, there is so far little evidence that Type IV reactions are implicated in either acute or chronic urticaria.

Finally, anaphylatoxins derived from the activated third and fifth components of the complement and known to produce histamine release from mast cells, may be responsible for some of the so far unidentified cases of chronic urticaria.[114–116]

Clinical features

Examination of the skin reveals a raised red weal with a whitish centre which might not be initially obvious. The distribution and size of the weals vary but they are usually between 2 and 5 mm in diameter. Occasionally very large weals are seen and bullae may form in their centres. Most commonly such weals are seen on the legs. At times urticarial lesions develop in very particular sites of the body such as on the exposed areas following sunburn or on areas subjected to the pressure of a garment (Cobner phenomenon).

The natural history of the weal is for it to last for a number of hours but to clear up completely in about 48 hours. Large lesions may last for two to four days and moderate itching is then present. This is especially prominent when urticaria involves the face, hands and feet. Itching is usually absent in cases or urticaria which have developed subcutaneous extension (angioedema). In angioedema, swellings which may involve any part of the body develop rapidly. Such swellings are most commonly seen on the face, especially round the eyes and lips, but also other organs such as tongue, palate or even the larynx. Such symptoms however are more often associated with hereditary angioedema.

Once an urticarial rash completely clears up, the skin may occasionally show some purpuric spots, especially if there has been a fair amount of itching. It is unusual for the same site to be involved within hours or even days. Broadly speaking, large or odd shaped weals occur in acute states and small weals in chronic episodes of urticaria. The same is possibly true in instances of food allergy when variable weals are present. Not uncommonly albuminuria of a transient nature is present during acute attacks, although serious renal complications are occasionally seen following serum sickness. In such instances urticarial rash develops between six and ten days following administration of the noxious substance. Features will vary from a mild generalised anaphylactic reaction or there may be a rapid onset of shock-like state. Cardiac complications such as ECG changes and pain are uncommon and cerebral oedema is extremely rare.

Differential diagnosis

Although in the majority of cases, diagnosis of urticaria is fairly straightforward, occasionally difficulties may arise. Urticaria should be differentiated from atopic dermatitis and other causes of eczema. The most common source of confusion is insect bites and stings. In such instances, history and close examination of the skin is essential. Typically papular lesions will be seen and are due to an allergic reaction to the saliva of the biting insect. Biphasic reactions (Type I and Type IV) are observed in such cases (as commonly occurs with heat lumps). This is clinically important and will give an important clue to the correct diagnosis.

Schonlein–Henoch Syndrome. Although many children will show purpuric lesions some may initially start with urticarial eruptions. The characteristic distribution of lesions on legs, buttocks and extensor surfaces of the arms and involvement of large joints, gastrointestinal tract and the kidneys will point to the right diagnosis.

Erythema marginatum. Easily distinguished by its appearance of ring patterns and the absence of itching. There will be other features of rheumatic fever.

Erythema multiforme. Has a characteristic clinical appearance (target lesions) and in doubtful cases can be distinguished from urticaria on histological grounds. A child who presents with erythema multiforme should be suspected of having rheumatoid arthritis. It is useful to remember that such a rash may precede the onset of arthritis by many months.

Urticaria pigmentosa (mastocytosis). Due to localised infiltrations of mast cells in the skin. Weals may occur following trauma, drugs or spontaneously. If areas (nodules) of mast cells are saturated or rubbed a weal will develop (Darier's sign). Once a weal has subsided the underlying pigmentation will of course persist. Other organs may be affected.

The differential diagnosis of angioedema is from hereditary angioedema, contact dermatitis, acute infection, the Melkersson–Rosenthal Syndrome[117,118] (cause unknown, recurrent swelling of the lips, facial palsy, tendency to residual thickening of the tissues), very rarely idiopathic scrotal oedema,[119] and superior vena cava obstruction which may occasionally present with recurrent swelling of the face.[120]

Hereditary angioedema.[121,122] This condition should be excluded in any child who presents with angioedema. There may be positive family history. It is transmitted as an autosmal dominant, boys and girls being equally affected. Clinical features and severity of attacks are variable but may involve the subcutaneous tissues of any site of the body. In young children the gastrointestinal tract is often affected giving rise to recurrent abdominal pain or colic in the very young baby. Involvement of the larynx may lead to fatal asphyxia. Diagnosis is established by estimating C1 esterase inhibitor by esterolytic technique.[121] Treatment consists of regular administration of E-aminocaproic acid (EACA)[123,124] or tranexamic acid,[125] fresh plasma for acute attacks[126] or before surgical procedures.[129] There is a mortality of 20–30 per cent.[127]

It is also worth remembering that some children with angioedema and papular eruptions have been found to have normal serum values of C1 esterase inhibitor but reduced concentrations of $C1_2$, C4 and C2.[128]

Investigations

These are rarely required in acute urticaria. In chronic states, a white cell count should be performed as a high eosonophil count would suggest allergy or a parasitic infestation. Serum immunoglobulins and IgE levels are normal in both acute and chronic urticaria. Any focus of chronic infection should be excluded by the appropriate investigations. Allergy skin tests may occasionally be helpful. More specialised tests such as the determinations of the serum C1 esterase inhibitor, other components of the complement, cryoglobulins and skin biopsy would be dictated by the history. Challenge tests with suspected foods have only limited practical value.

Management

In the majority of cases, urticaria is a self limiting condition requiring very little active treatment. A detailed history may pinpoint a specific cause or factor. The single most important advice during the acute stage is to discontinue any drugs, agents or other unusual foods which the child might have been taking. A detailed daily record card should be kept if urticaria occurs frequently.

Episodes of solar urticaria may be considerably reduced by graded exposure to sunlight, avoidance of strong sun rays and topical administration of some skin barrier agents such as maxenon and titanium dioxide creams (for long wave lengths) or 5 per cent *p*-aminosalicylic acid preparations.[135] The use of long-term chlorquine in children is not justified.[136] Cold urticaria is helped by avoiding cold baths, drinks, etc. and responds very well to antihistamines (see Table 5.5). The beneficial value of large doses of penicillin has been documented in adults but not in children.[137] Cholinergic urticaria (exercise, emotion, temperature changes) respond to cool baths following attacks, ultraviolet light[138] and occasionally hypnosis.

Antihistamines. Despite their many side effects, antihistamines occupy an important place in the management of urticaria. They act by occupying the receptor sites of the receptor cells to the exclusion of histamine. They have widespread properties and actions such as antiserotonin, antiadrenaline and anticholinergic effects, and they cause depression of the central nervous system which accounts for the majority of the side-effects. There is little to choose between the various antihistamines currently available. However, about 20 per cent of children with acute or chronic urticaria will not respond to antihistamines.

The beneficial effects of antihistamines will as a rule be produced within 1 hour of administration and the peak effect being reached at about 3 hours. By 8 to 12 hours at least 50 per cent of the drug will have been excreted. Tolerance to antihistamines varies from child to child but should be suspected after one or two months treatment. The Table 5.5 describes some of the antihistamines used in urticaria.

Table 5.5

Antihistamine	Daily dose (mg/kg)
Hydroxyzine	2
Cyprohepatidine	0·25
Piphenlydromine	5
Promethazine	2
Brompheniramine valerate	0·4

Corticosteroids. In general these are not required either in acute or chronic urticaria but may be used in severe cases especially in serum sickness.

Hyposensitisation. No studies have been published which convincingly prove that specific hyposensitisation is of value in chronic urticaria.

Other drugs. Sedation may occasionally be required. The beneficial value of heparin,[130] calcium,[131] trasylol,[132] and indomethacin[133] remains unproven. However, the use of beta$_2$ adrenergic stimulants in chronic urticaria is most promising.[134,135,139]

Other agents. Subcutaneous injection of 1:1000 adrenaline 0·5–1 ml should always be considered in cases of acute urticaria associated with angioedema swellings. This is especially important when the oedema involves the throat and lips. If such conditions recur frequently long-term ephedrine sulphate or sublingual isoprenaline sulphate (for the older child) is worth considering.

References

1. Rajka, G. (1975) *Atopic Dermatitis.* Philadelphia: W. B. Saunders.
2. Prose, P. H. (1965) Pathologic changes in eczema. *J. Pediatr.,* **66,** 178.
3. Scott, A. (1958) The distribution and behaviour of cutaneous nerves in normal and abnormal skin. *Br. J. Dermatol.,* **70,** 1.
4. Ash, A. S. F. and Schild, H. O. (1966) Receptors mediating some actions of histamine. *Br. J. Pharmacol.,* **27,** 427.
5. Greaves, N. W., Sondergaard, J. and McDonald-Gibson, W. (1971) Recovery of prostaglandins in cutaneous inflammation. *Br. med. J.,* **II,** 258.
6. Pasternack, B. (1965) The prediction of asthma in infantile eczema. *J. Pediatr.,* **66,** 164.
7. Walker, R. B. and Warin, R. P. (1956) The incidence of eczema in early childhood. *Br. J. Dermatol.,* **68,** 182.
8. Stifler, W. C. (1965) A 21 year follow-up of infantile eczema. *J. Pediatr.,* **66,** 166.
9. Liddell, K., (1976) A familial study of acne and eczema. *Br. J. Dermatol.,* **94,** 633.
10. Wheatley, V. R. (1965) Secretions of the skin in eczema. *J. Pediatr.,* **66,** 200.
11. Vowles, M., Warin, R. P. and Appley, J. (1955) Infantile eczema: observations on natural history and prognosis. *Br. J. Dermatol.,* **67,** 53.
12. Musgrove, K. and Morgan, J. K. (1976) Infantile eczema: A long-term follow up study. *Br. J.Dermatol.,* **95,** 365.
13. Norins, A. L. (1971) Atopic dermatitis. *Pediatr. Clin. N. Am.,* **18,** 801.
14. Rajka, G. (1960) Prurigo Besnier (atopic dermatitis) with special reference to the role of allergic factors. *Acta dermato-venereolog.,* **40,** 285.
15. Rajka, G. (1961) Atopic dermatitis. *Acta dermato-venereolog.,* **41,** 363.
16. Sneddon, I. (1967) Treatment of atopic eczema. In: *Treatment of Common Skin Diseases.* p. 31, London: British Medical Association.
17. Davis, L. R., Marten, R. H. and Sarkany, I. (1961) Atopic eczema in European and negro West Indian infants in London. *Br. J. Dermatol.,* **73,** 410.
18. Worth, R. M. (1962) Atopic dermatitis among Chinese infants in Honolulu and San Francisco. *Hawaii med. J.,* **22,** 31.
19. Juhlin, L., Johansson, S. G. O., Bennich, H., Hogman, C. and Thyresson, N. (1969) Immunoglobulin E in dermatoses levels in atopic dermatitis and urticaria. *Archs Dermatol.,* **100,** 12.
20. Johansson, S. G. O. and Juhlin, L. (1970) Immunoglobulin E in 'healed' atopic dermatitis and after treatment with corticosteroids and azathoprine. *Br. J. Dermatol.,* **82,** 10.
21. Stone, S. P., Gleich, G. J. and Muller, S. A. (1976) Atopic dermatitis and IgE. Relationship between changes in IgE levels and severity of the disease. *Archs. Dermatol.,* **112,** 1254.

22. Parish, W. E. and Champion, R. H. (1973) Atopic dermatitis. In: *Recent Advances in Dermatology*. Ed. by Rook, A., p. 143. Edinburgh: Churchill-Livingstone.
23. Winkelmann, R. K. (1966) Non-allergic factors in atopic dermatitis. *J. Allergy*, **37**, 29.
24. Sly, R. M. and Heimlich, E. M. (1967) Physiologic abnormalities in the atopic state: a review. *Annls Allergy.*, **25**, 192.
25. Berrens, L. (1970) The allergens in house dust. *Progr. Allergy*, **14**, 259.
26. Winkelmann, R. K., Johnson, L. A. and West, J. R. (1962) Delayed blanch phenomenon in atopic individuals without dermatitis. *Archs Dermatol.*, **85**, 222.
27. Champion, R. H. (1963) Abnormal vascular reactions in atopic eczema. *Br. J. Dermatol.*, **75**, 12.
28. Olive, J. T., O'Connell, E. J. and Winkelmann, R. K. (1970) Delayed blanch phenomen in children; re-evaluation of 5 year old children originally tested as newborns. *J. Invest. Dermatol.*, **54**, 356.
29. Brystryn, J. C. and Hyman, C. (1969) Skin blood flow in atopic dermatitis. *J. Invest. Dermatol.*, **52**, 189.
30. Stenius, B., Wide, L. and Seymour, W. M. (1972) Clinical significance of total IgE and of specific IgE to *Dermatophagoides*, spp., grass pollen and other common allergens. *Clin. Allergy*, **2**, 303.
31. Warndorff, J. A. (1970) The response of the sweat gland to acetylcholine in atopic subjects. *Br. J. Dermatol.*, **83**, 306.
32. Hansen, A. E., Haggard, M. E., Boelsche, A. N., Adam, D. J. D. and Weise, M. F. (1958) Essential fatty acids in infant nutrition—III. Clinical manifestations of linoleic acid deficiencies. *J. Nutri.*, **66**, 565.
33. Caldwell, M. D., Jonsson, H. T. and Othersen, H. B. (1972) Essential fatty acid deficiency in an infant receiving prolonged parenteral alimentation. *J. Pediatr.*, **81**, 894.
34. Prottey, C. (1976) Essential fatty acids and the skin. *Brit. J. Dermatol.*, **94**, 579.
35. Savin, J. A., Paterson, W. D. and Oswald, I. (1973) Scratching during sleep. *Lancet*, **II**, 296.
36. Savin, J. A., Paterson, W. D., Oswald, I. and Adam, K. (1975) Further studies of scratching during sleep. *Br. J. Dermatol.*, **93**, 297.
37. Rajka, G. (1967) Itch duration in the involved skin of atopic dermatitis. *Acta dermato-venereolog.*, **47**, 154.
38. Jacobs, J. C. and Miller, M. E. (1972) Fatal familial Leiner's disease: A deficiency of the opsonic activity of serum complement. *Pediatrics*, **49**, 225.
39. Miller, M. E. and Koblenzer, P. J. (1972) Leiner's disease and deficiency of C5. *J. Pediatr.*, **80**, 879.
40. Rosenfeld, S. I. and Leddy, J. P. (1974) Hereditary deficiency of the fifth component of complement. *J. clin. Invest.*, **53**, 67a.
41. Blume, B. R. and Wolff, S. M. (1972) Chediak-Higashi. Review and report of new patients. *Medicine*, **51**, 247.
42. Belohralski, B. H., Finstad, J. and Fudenberg, H. H. (1974) Primary immunodeficiency diseases in man (workshops). *Clin. Immunol. Immunopathol.*, **2**, 281.
43. Rosen, F. S. (1976) The primary immunodeficiencies: Dermatologic manifestations. *J. invest. Dermatol.*, **67**, 402.
44. Hill, H. R., Quie, P. G., Pabst, H. F. (1974) Defect in neutrophil granulocyte chemotaxis in Job's Syndrome of recurrent 'cold' staphylococcal abcesses. *Lancet*, **II**, 617.
45. Thompson, E. N. and Soothill, J. F. (1970) Chronic granulomatous disease—quantitative clinicopathological relationship. *Archs dis. Child.*, **45**, 24.
46. Reed, W. B., Epstein, W. L., Boder, E. and Sedgewick, R. (1966) Cutaneous manifestations of ataxia-telangiectasia. *J. Am. med. Ass.*, **195**, 746.
47. Weary, P. E., Manley, W. F. and Graham, G. F. (1972) Hereditary acrokeratotic poikiloderma. *Archs Dermatol.*, **103**, 409.

48. Reed, W. B., Lopez, D. A. and Landing, B. (1970) Clinical spectrum of anhidrotic ectodermal dysplasia. *Archs Dermatol.*, **102,** 134.
49. Peterson, R. D. A. (1965) Immunologic responses in infantile eczema. *J. Pediatr.*, **66,** 224.
50. Oppenheim, J. J., Blaese, R. M. and Waldmann, T. A. (1970) Defective lymphocyte transformation and delayed sensitivity in Wiskott–Aldrich Syndrome. *Proc. nat. Acad. Sci.*, **66,** 1119.
51. Blaese, R. M., Strober, W., Brown, R. S. and Waldmann, T. A. (1968) The Wiskott–Aldrich Syndrome. *Lancet*, **I,** 1056.
52. Soloman, L. M. and Esterly, N. B. (1973) *Neonatal Dermatology*, p. 130. Philadelphia: W. B. Saunders.
53. Johnston, R. B. and Newman, S. L. (1977) Chronic granulomatous disease. *Pediatr. Clin. N. Am.*, **24,** 2, 365.
54. Barnett, H. L. and Einhorn, A. H. (1972) *Pediatrics*. 15th ed. p. 324. New York: Appleton–Century–Crofts.
55. Snyderman, S. E., Boyer, A., Roctmann, E., Holt, L. E. and Prose, P. H. (1963) The histidine requirement of the infant. *Pediatrics*, **31,** 786.
56. Insley, J. (1967) Syndrome associated with a deficiency of part of the long arms of chromosome No. 18. *Archs dis. Child.*, **42,** 140.
57. Smith, D. W. (1970) *Recognisable Patterns of Human Malformation*, p. 50. Philadelphia: W. B. Saunders.
58. Pincus, S. H., Thomas, I. T., Clark, R. A. and Ochs, H. D. (1975) Defective neutrophil chemotaxis with variant ichthyosis, hyperimmunoglobulinaemia E and recurrent infections. *J. Pediatr.*, **87,** 908.
59. Weston, W. L. (1977) Cutaneous manifestations of defective host defences. *Pediatr. Clin. N. Am.*, **24,** 2, 395.
60. Behrens, M. M. (1974) Optic atrophy in children after diiodohydroxymine therapy. *J. Am. med. Ass.*, **228,** 693.
61. Shuster, S. and Marks, J. (1965) Dermatogenic enteropathy: a new cause of steatorrhea. *Lancet*, **I,** 1367.
62. Bergsma, D., Ed. (1972) *Birth Defects—Atlas and Compendium*. Baltimore: Williams and Wilkins.
63. Grosse, R., Gorlin, J. and Opitz, J. M. (1971) The Dubowitz Syndrome. *Z. Kinderheilk*, **110,** 175.
64. Krueger, G. G., Kahn, G., Weston, W. L. and Mandel, M. J. (1973) IgE levels in nummular eczema and ichthyosis. *Archs Dermatol.*, **107,** 56.
65. Leyden, J. J., Marples, R. R. and Kligman, A. M. (1974) Staphylococcus aureus in the lesions of atopic dermatitis. *Br. J. Dermatol.*, **90,** 525.
66. Higgins, P. G. and Crow, K. D. (1973) Coxsackie virus A16 in Kaposi's eruption. *Brit. J. Dermatol.*, **88,** 391.
67. Gottlieb, B. R. and Hanifin, J. M. (1974) Circulating T cell deficiency in atopic dermatitis. *Clin. Res.*, **23,** 159a.
68. Copeman, P. W. M. and Wallace, H. J. (1964) Eczema vaccinatum. *Br. med. J.*, **2,** 906.
69. Grosfield, J. C. M. and van Ramshorst, A. G. S. (1970) Eczema vaccinatum. *Dermatologica* **141,** 1.
70. *Report of the Committee on Infectious Diseases* (1974), 17th ed., p. 163 American Academy of Pediatrics.
71. Kaufman H. and Roth H. (1974) Hyposensitisation with alum precipitated extracts in atopic dermatitis: A placebo controlled study. *Annls Allergy*, **32,** 321.
72. Jacobs, A. H. (1972) Management of children with atopic dermatitis. *Cutis*, **10,** 585.
73. Scholtz, J. R. (1965) Management of atopic dermatitis. *Cal. Med.*, **102,** 210.
74. Du Vivier, A. and Stoughton, R. B. (1975) Tachyphylaxis to the action of topically applied corticosteroids. *Archs Dermatol.*, **111,** 581.
75. Staughton, R. C. D. and August, P. J. (1975) Cushing's Syndrome and pituitary–adrenal suppression due to clobetasol propionate. *Br. med. J.*, **II,** 419.

76. Du Vivier, A. and Stoughton, R. B. (1976) Acute tolerance to the effects of topical glucocorticosteroids. *Br. J. Dermatol.*, **94**, Suppl. 12, 25.
77. Carruthers, J. A., August, P. J. and Staughton, R. C. D. (1975) Observations on the systemic effect of topical clobetasol propionate. *Br. med. J.*, **IV**, 203.
78. Munro, D. D. and Wilson, L. (1975) Clobetasone butyrate. A new topical corticosteroid: Clinical activity and effects on pituitary adrenal axis function and model of epidermal atrophy. *Br. med. J.*, **III**. 626.
79. Greaves, M. S. (1971) The *in vivo* catabolism of cortisol by human skin. *J. invest. Dermatol.*, **57**, 100.
80. Feiwel, M., Munro, D. D. and James, V. H. T. (1968) Effect of topically applied 0·1% betamethasone 17-valerate ointment on the adrenal function of children. In: XIII *Congressus Internationalis Dermatologial*. Ed. by Jodassohn, W. and Schirren, C. G., Vol. 1, p. 202. Berlin: Springer.
81. Kirby, J. D. and Munro, D. D. (1976) Steroid-induced atrophy in an animal and human model. *Br. J. Dermatol.*, **94**, suppl. 12, 111.
82. Sneddon, I. B. (1976) Atropy of the skin. The clinical problems. *Br. J. Dermatol.*, **94**, suppl. 12, 121.
83. Kuzemko, J. A. and Bedford, S. (1976) *Asthma in Children*, p. 62. Tunbridge Wells: Pitman Medical.
84. Magnusson, B. and Kligman, A. M. (1970) Identification of contact allergens. In: *Contact Dermatitis in the Guinea Pig*, p. 102. Springfield: Charles C. Thomas.
85. Coombs, R. R. A. and Gell, P. G. H. (1975) In: *Clinical Aspects of Immunology*. Ed. by Gell, P. G. H., Coombs, R. R. H. and Lachmann, P. J., p. 778. Oxford: Blackwell Scientific.
86. Goldyne, M. E., Winklemann, R. K. and Ryan, R. J. (1973) Prostaglandin activity in human cutaneous inflammation detection by radioimmunoassay. *Prostaglandins*, **4**, 737.
87. Lowe, N. J., Virgadamo, F. and Stoughton, R. B. (1977) Anti-inflammatory properties of a prostaglandin antagonist, a corticosteroid and indomethacin in experimental contact dermatitis. *Br. J. Dermatol.*, **96**, 433.
88. Medenica, M. and Rostenberg, A. (1971) Comparative and electron microscopic study of primary irritant contact dermatitis and allergic contact dermatitis. *J. invest. Dermatol.*, **56**, 259.
89. Milliken, L. E., Conway, F. and Foote, J. E. (1973) *In vitro* studies of contact hypersensitivity: lymphocyte transformation in nickel sensitivity. *J. invest. Dermatol.*, **60**, 88.
90. Nishioka, K. and Amos, H. E. (1972) Contact sensitivity *in vitro*. *Trans. St John's Hosp. Dermatol. Soc.*, **58**, 142.
91. Levene, G. M. (1972) Lymphocyte transformation in contact sensitivity. *Trans. St John's Hosp. Dermatol. Soc.*, **58**, 147.
92. Rostenberg, A. and Solomon, L. M. (1968) Jean Hein Fabre and the patch test. *Archs Dermatol.*, **98**, 188.
93. Coudie, M. W. and Adams, R. M. (1973) Influence of oral prednisone on patch test reactions Rhus antigens. *Archs Dermatol.*, **107**, 540.
94. Cronin, E. (1972) Clinical prediction of patch test results. *Trans. St John's Hosp. Dermatol. Soc.*, **58**, 153.
95. Fisher, A. A. (1969) *Contact Dermatitis*. London: Kimpton.
96. Haider, S. A. (1977) Treatment of atopic eczeme in children: Clinical trial of 10% sodium cromoglycate ointment. *Br. med. J.*, **I**, 1570.
97. Jacobs, A. H. (1969) Local management of atopic dermatitis in infants and children. *Clin. Pediatrics*, **8**, 201.
98. Harber, L. C., Harris, H. and Baer, R. L. (1966) Photoallergic contact dermatitis. *Archs Dermatol.*, **94**, 255.
99. Bendkowski, B. (1968) Urticaria. *Curr. Med. Drugs*, **8**, 11.
100. Hellgren, L. (1972) The prevalence of urticaria in the total population. *Acta allerg.*, **27**, 2, 36.

101. Sheldon, J. M., Matthews, K. P. and Lovell, R. G. (1954) The vexing urticaria problem. Present concepts of aetiology and management. *J. Allergy*, **25**, 525.
102. Moore-Robinson, M. and Warin, R. P. (1968) Some clinical aspects of cholinergic urticaria. *Br. J. Dermatol.*, **80**, 794.
103. Kuzemko, J. A. (1977) Unpublished data.
104. Warin, R. P. and Champion, R. H. (1974) *Urticaria*, p. 13. Philadelphia: W. B. Saunders.
105. Champion, R. H., Roberts, S. O. B., Carpenter, R. G. and Roger, J. H. (1969) Urticaria and angioedema. *Br. J. Dermatol.*, **81**, 588.
106. Matthews, K. P. (1974) A current view of urticaria. *Med. Clin. N. Am.*, **58**, 189.
107. Hellgen, L. and Hersle, K. (1964) Acute and chronic urticaria. *Acta allerg.*, **19**, 406.
108. Kjellman, M. N. I. (1976) *Immunolobulin E and Atopic Allergy in Childhood*. Linköping University Medical Dissertations No. 36. Linköping.
109. Buckley, R. H. and Dees, S. C. (1967) Serum immunoglobulins. Abnormalities associated with chronic urticaria in children. *J. Allergy*, **40**, 294.
110. Rogge, J. L. and Hanifin, J. M. (1976) Immunodeficiencies in severe atopic dermatitis. *Archs Dermatol.*, **112**, 1391.
111. Mines, S. C., Levine, M. I. and Fireman, P. (1969) Serum immunogloublin levels in acute and chronic urticaria. *J. Allergy*, **44**, 20.
112. Snyderman, R.,Rogers, E. and Buckley, R. H. (1977) Abnormalities of leukotaxis in atopic dermatitis. *J. Allergy Clin. Immunol.*, **60**, 121.
113. Cream, J. J. and Turk, J. L. (1971) A review of the evidence for immune complex deposition as a cause of skin disease in man. *Clin. Allergy*, **1**, 235.
114. DeSilva, W. D. and Lepow, I. H. (1967) Complement as a mediator of inflammation, Biological properties of anaphylatoxins prepared with purified components of complement. *J. exp. Med.*, **125**, 921.
115. Whepper, K. D., Bokisch, V. A., Müller-Eberhard, H. J. and Stoughton, R. B. (1972) Cutaneous responses for human C_3 anaphylatoxin in man. *Clin. exp. Immunol.*, **11**, 13.
116. Lachman, P. J. (1975) Complement. In: *Clinical Aspects of Immunology*. Ed. by Gell, P. G. H., Coombs, R. R. A. and Lachman, P. J., 3rd ed, p. 341. Oxford: Blackwell Scientific.
117. Kettel, K. (1947) Melkersson's Syndrome. *Archs Orolaryngol.*, **46**, 341.
118. Pindborg, J. J. (1972) Disorders of the oral cavity and lips. In: *Textbook of Dermatology*. Ed. by Rook, A. J., Wilkinson, D. S. and Ebling, F. J., 2nd ed. chap. 57. Oxford: Blackwell Scientific.
119. Hanstead, B. and John, H. T. (1964) Idiopathic scrotal oedema of children. *Br. J. Urol.*, **36**, 110.
120. Mancher, O. M. and Burgard, W. (1973) Pseudo-quincke Odem als Ansdruck einer oberen Einflusstanung, *Hantarzt*, **24**, 39.
121. Hadjiyannaki, K. and Lachmann, P. J. (1971) Hereditary angioedema: A review with particular reference to pathogenisis and treatment. *Clin. Allergy*, **1**, 221.
122. Bedford, S. and Kuzemko, J. A. (1971) Hereditary angio-oedema. *Proc. R. Soc. Med.*, **64**, 1049.
123. Champion, R. H., Roberts, S. O. B., Carpenter, R. and Roger, J. (1969) Hereditary angioedema treated with E-aminocaproic acid. *Br. J. Dermatol.*, **81**, 763.
124. Frank, M. M., Sergeant, J. S., Kane, M. A. and Alling, D. W. (1972) Epsilon aminocaproic acid therapy of hereditary angioneurotic oedema. A double blind study. *New Eng. Med. J.*, **286**, 808.
125. Sheffer, A. L., Austen, K. F. and Rosen, F. S. (1972) Tranexamic acid therapy in hereditary angioedema. *New Eng. Med. J.*, **287**, 452.
126. Pickering, R. J., Kelly, J. R., Good, R. A. and Gewurz, H. (1969) Replacement therapy in hereditary angioedema. Successful treatment of two patients with fresh frozen plasma. *Lancet*, **I**, 326.
127. Austen, K. H. and Sheffer, A. L. (1965) Detection of hereditary angioneurotic oedema by demonstration of a reduction in the second component of human comple-

ment. *New Eng. Med. J.*, **272**, 649.

128. Sissons, J. G. P., Williams, D. G., Peters, D. K. and Boulton Jones, J. M. (1974) Skin lesions, angioedema and hypocomplementaemia. *Lancet*, **II**, 1350.

129. Jaffe, C. J. (1975) Hereditary angioedema: the use of fresh frozen plasma for prophylaxis in patients undergoing oral surgery. *J. Allergy Clin. Immunol.*, **55**, 386.

130. Thompson, J. S. (1968) Urticaria and angioedema. *Ann. intern. Med.*, **69**, 361.

131. Parker, W. (1950) Clinical observations in the use of combined calcium-antihistamine therapy in the treatment of urticaria. *Annls Allergy*, **8**, 765.

132. Berova, N. (1974) In: *Urticaria*. Ed. by Warin, R. P. and Champion, R. H., p. 109. Philadelphia: W. B. Saunders.

133. Zacharial, H., Niordson, A. M. and Hemingsen, S. J. (1969) Indemthacin in urticaria and histamine induced wealing. *Acta dermato-venereolog.*, **49**, 49.

134. Kram, J., Bourne, H., Maibach, H. and Melmon, K. (1975) Cutaneous immediate hypersensitivity in man. Effects of systematically administered adrenergic drugs. *J. Allergy Clin. Immunol.*, **56**, 387.

135. Macleod, T. M. and Frain-Bell, W. (1971) The study of the efficacy of some agents used for the protection of the skin from exposure to light. *Br. J. Dermatol.*, **84**, 266.

136. Shapiro, A. L. (1967) How I treat physical urticaria. *Postgrad. Med.*, **41**, 147.

137. Obermayer, M. E. (1963) Treatment of cold urticaria with penicillin. *Archs Dermatol.*, **87**, 269.

138. Garretts, M. (1958) Cholinergic urticaria and miliaria. *Br. J. Dermatol.*, **70**, 166.

139. Kennes, B., DeMaubeuge, J. and Delespesse, G. (1977) Treatment of chronic urticaria with beta$_2$-adrenergic stimulant. *Clin. Allergy*, **7**, 35.

CHAPTER 6

Allergic Disease of the Upper Respiratory Tract

ALTHOUGH THE PRIMITIVE function of the nose is olfactory, the nasal apparatus possesses other important actions such as heat regulation, humidification of inspired air and protection against infections. Little is known about the importance and course of ingoing and outgoing air-streams, of nasal secretions, of the autonomic nerve supply of the nasal mucosa, ciliary function and the effects of various drugs on the normal physiological activities. Similarly the function of the sinuses remains undetermined.[1-3]

It is against such background that allergic disorders of the upper respiratory tract in children should be considered. They are common but often mis-diagnosed as recurrent colds, infections or more liberally as catarrh. In one study of 100 toddlers, it was found that in 70 the 'recurrent colds' were in fact episodes of allergic rhinitis.[4] Classification of rhinitis in some of the standard paediatric textbooks if often vague and confusing. The following is the scheme we use:

Rhinitis

a. *Acute*   Infective (virus, bacteria)
                              Allergic

b. *Chronic:*

     1. Allergic   Seasonal (pollenosis or hay fever).
                              Perennial (non-seasonal)

     2. Vasomotor   Physical agents, e.g. sudden change of temperature.
                              Mechanical, e.g. dust, smoke, foreign body.
                              Psychosomatic.

     3. Infective   'Post-nasal drip', T.B., sarcoid.

     4. Iatrogenic   Nasal drips and sprays.
                              Hypotensive agents.

     5. Specific   Congenital anomalies, hypothyroidism.

Incidence

The prevalence of seasonal and perennial allergic rhinitis has been estimated as between 2 and 20 per cent.[6-9] There is little doubt that allergic rhinitis is much more common than is realised. About 5 per cent of children with pollenosis will eventually develop asthma.[5,37] Pollenosis is more common in boys, it often starts at around 4 to 6 years of age and symptoms may occur between 2 and 25 seasons. Perennial rhinitis is more common in boys and in 30 per cent symptoms persist into adult life. The peak incidence occurs in early adolescence and the duration of symptoms varies between 2 and 15 years.[9,38] Skin sensitivity tests in this group of children often show positive reactions to many allergens and nasal eosinophilia is found in over 50 per cent and especially in those sensitive to cats, dogs, grass pollens and house dust.[20]

Immunological aspects

The child who is genetically predisposed to develop atopic disease becomes sensitised by inhalation or ingestion of antigens during early life. Following such frequent exposure the antigens react with specific IgE antibody on the surface of mast cells which cluster around the nasal epithelium. Type I immediate reaction occurs leading to the release of the various chemical mediators and thus production of symptoms such as excessive mucous, itching and nasal blockage. Undoubtedly histamine is one of the major mediators concerned,[13] but other agents such as kinins may be responsible for the increased capillary permeability and vasodilation which occurs, and the eosinophilic chemotactic factor of anaphylaxis is very probably involved in attracting clusters of eosinophils to the nasal mucosa.[10-12] Some of these changes can be demonstrated following biopsy specimen during exacerbations.[14,16,23] In some children repeated allergen exposure may lead to the reduction in the allergen challenge threshold of mucosa so that even low atmospheric allergen counts may still result in symptoms.[15] Such an effect may persist for several weeks and also lower the threshold for other allergens which normally do not cause any symptoms. This is worth bearing in mind for example in the child with persistent symptoms after the end of the official pollen season.

It has also been shown that individuals sensitive to grass pollens may develop both immediate and late nasal reactions.[18] During the immediate reaction which lasts for about an hour the subject develops some nasal discharge and sneezing. During the late reaction which occurs 4 to 6 hours following challenge signs of nasal obstruction develop. There is some histological evidence that nasal blocking is due to the increase in goblet cells and thus production of thick mucus.[17]

Diagnosis

Seasonal symptoms

a. Sudden and recurrent episodes of sneezing and itching inside the nose.
b. Variable watery nasal discharge.
c. Partial or complete nasal obstruction.
d. Associated watering of the eyes with itching and often swelling of the eyelids due to constant rubbing of the eyes.

Perennial symptoms

These may be similar to those of seasonal allergic rhinitis but are usually much less acute and the eyes are rarely involved. Onset of symptoms is sudden and the episode may continue unabated for a few hours or two or three days. Some children may complain of headache, pain over the paranasal sinuses, a dry throat or a repetitive cough which is due to the drainage of the nasal mucus into the posterior pharynx. Irritation of the larynx may cause hoarseness. Infrequent bouts of vomiting may occur due to the swallowing of large amounts of mucus.

Physical signs

Nasal mucosa appears bluish and pale although immediately following an attack it may be reddish and intensely engorged. The inferior turbinates are enlarged and nasal obstruction is due to their engorgement. Inspection of the floor of the nostrils often reveals oedema of the turbinates which are covered with mucoid discharge. This contributes further to the nasal obstruction, and inevitably leads to mouth breathing. The lack of nose breathing may also contribute to the degree of nasal obstruction which may be aggravated by temperature changes or supine posture.[19] At times it can be very difficult to distinguish such changes from vasomotor rhinitis but other features of allergy will often be present.

Some of the facial characteristics of allergic rhinitis have been fully described previously on pages 24–26. Figure 6.1 illustrates some of the features:

Allergic rhinitis should be distinguished from vasomotor rhinitis which shows generalised thickening of the nasal mucosa involving the septum and the turbinates, the thickening being especially marked over the inferior turbinates. The mucosa is often reddish and soggy. Post nasal mirror examination shows gross thickening of the posterior nares and turbinates on each side. These are pale grey in colour and may block the posterior nares. At times an enlargement of the posterior end of the in-

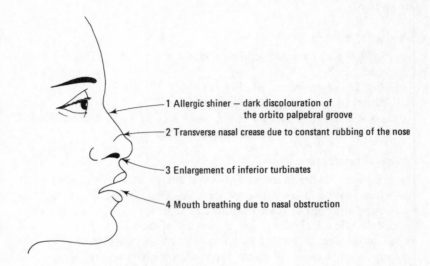

1 Allergic shiner – dark discolouration of
the orbito palpebral groove

2 Transverse nasal crease due to constant rubbing of the nose

3 Enlargement of inferior turbinates

4 Mouth breathing due to nasal obstruction

Fig. 6.1 Facial characteristics of allergic rhinitis. 1—allergic shiner, dark discoloration of the orbitopalpebral groove; 2—Transverse nasal crease due to constant rubbing of the nose upwards (allergic salute); 3—Enlargement of inferior turbinates; 4—Mouth breathing due to nasal obstruction.

ferior turbinates is seen which is practically never seen in allergic rhinitis. The distinction from infectious rhinitis is fairly straightforward (fever, some degree of constitutional upset, thick and discoloured discharge, absent family history of atopy and nasal neutrophilia).

Investigations

The blood eosinophil count may be raised ($300/mm^3$). Examination of nasal secretions will often demonstrate between 5 and 10 per cent eosinophils. However, in a child under the age of 1 year nasal eosinophilia should be interpreted with caution as this may be a normal finding.[21,22] Absence of eosinophils in the nasal secretions does not exclude allergic rhinitis, especially in those children in whom it is complicated by a nonspecific infection. There is also some evidence that in some children who develop rhinitis due to food allergy, nasal eosinophilia may be absent.[22]

Skin sensitivity tests to various allergens are often positive and correlate well with history, nasal provocation tests and specific serum IgE values as determined by the radioallergosorbent method (RAST). Analysis of nasal secretions for specific IgE antibodies is of little practical value.[24,25] These investigations should be performed because they offer confirmatory evidence of allergy when one is considering a course of hyposensitisation and so that sound practical advice can be offered to the family regarding the avoidance of any possible precipitating factors. It is important to remember that positive skin tests should be interpreted with caution and scepticism if there is negative clinical history, since 15 to 30 per cent of normal children may give positive reaction to grass pollens and D. pteronyssinus.[39,40]

X-rays of the sinuses often show thickened lining and diminished air space. Fluid levels are rarely seen.

Treatment

General measures

In perennial allergic rhinitis it is at times possible to avoid exposure to the allergen responsible for symptoms. Thus, if there is strong evidence of hypersensitivity to the house dust mite, advice should be offered on how to reduce the population of the mite in the child's home. The living rooms should be vacuum cleaned at least once a week and furniture cleaned with a slightly damp cloth. The child's bedroom should be vacuum cleaned at least twice a week and bedding of synthetic material only used. Pillows and sheets should be changed weekly, the mattress should be covered with a polythene envelope and turned weekly, and curtains should be of light, easily washable material. Although the majority of houses have some central heating in the bedrooms, some still use paraffin heaters. Not only are these dangerous if left unattended, but because they give off water vapour, they create ideal growth conditions for the mite. Hence, these should be forbidden. In addition bedding should be aired in direct sunlight as often as possible. Household pets should be shampooed periodically and kept under control. The prophylactic use of a non-toxic bactericidal and fungicidal spray (Paragerm AK) in controlling the house dust mite household population (Dermatophagoides spp.) is currently being investigated.[28] Food allergens responsible for symptoms should be avoided and use of drugs strictly limited as over-use may lead to exacerbation of rhinitis.

The child who suffers from pollenosis should be advised to sleep with the bedroom windows closed during the season, avoid playing in the grass and stay indoors when the grass is being mown.

Medical measures

a. *Sympathomimetic agents.* Nasal administration of sympathomimetic drugs has been used for many years in the young child with perennial rhinitis mainly to relieve the nasal stuffiness which often interferes with feeding. Sympathomimetic agents act on the alpha receptors of the smooth muscle of arterioles producing vasoconstriction and thus reduction in oedema. With prolonged use vasodilatation occurs (rebound phenomenon) requiring increasing dosages in order to produce any further vasoconstriction. Moreover, as with other local agents, ciliary activity is considerably impaired, especially when solutions of different pH's are used. The pH of nasal mucus is 7·0.

Application of sympathomimetic drugs as drops, inhalations or solutions should last not longer than 3 to 4 days. Ephedrine, a sympathomimetic amine of 0·5 or 1 per cent in normal saline, has withstood the test of time. Relief is obtained within 10 to 15 minutes and lasts for from 2 to 4 hours. Phenylephine or xylometazoline are equally effective and have more prolonged action.

b. *Antihistamines.* In both seasonal and perennial rhinitis, oral antihistamines bring relief in about 50 per cent of children. They are useful if symptoms are mild, if itching predominates and nasal obstruction is minimal. However, side-effects are common. Drowsiness during the day may cause problems at school and dryness of the mouth often leads to excessive thirst. Antihistamines, therefore, should be used with caution and they are best given in the evening. For a succinct list of common antihistamine agents, please see page 60.

c. *Sodium cromoglycate.* This agent has been shown to be useful in the treatment of both types of rhinitis. The drug can be administered as a fine powder delivered by an insufflator or as a 2 per cent solution in a non-pressurised metered dose spray which allows greater accuracy of unit dose size.[29-34] It should be administered ideally before the exposure to the allergens because it acts by preventing the release of the various chemical mediators from mast cells and it is thus not really effective following antigen challenge. If the powder is used, it should be administered three or four times daily into each nostril. With drops or sprays the frequency of dosage should be increased to between six and eight times daily.

In pollenosis the treatment should be started one week before the official pollen season commences and continued for a week after the season is fully over.

In perennial allergic rhinitis, the dosage and duration of treatment remains largely empirical but should be continued for at least four to six weeks before it is decided that relief of symptoms is minimal. A daily record card is most useful as from one to three weeks may elapse before response is obtained. Overall at least 60 per cent of children with seasonal

and perennial rhinitis obtain relief from the use of sodium cromoglycate.
The Table below summarises results:

Table 6.1   Sodium cromoglycate in seasonal and perennial rhinitis

Reference	Year	Type of rhinitis	No. of patients	% improve-ment	Remarks
30	1971	Seasonal	27	70	—
35	1971	Seasonal (grass) (pollen)	50	71	In a laboratory study of 37 subjects protection was obtained against antigen challenge for about 6 hr by 10 mg SCG powder
31	1971	Seasonal	22	72	—
48	1971	Seasonal (grass)	54	50	Children studied only
36	1975	Perennial	19	68	Decrease in nasal eosinophilia
33	1975	Perennial	30	80	Double blind trial. Significant reduction in nasal eosinophilia. Five patients complained of nasal irritation on SCG
34	1977	Seasonal (grass)	44	100	Double blind trial. Spray used. Minimal nasal irritation in 3 patients

d. *Corticosteroids.* Systemic corticosteroids have been used for many
years in the treatment of seasonal allergic rhinitis in adults with some
success.[41,42] However, the relief of symptoms is relatively brief and the
frequent and often high doses required lead to side-effects including
adrenal suppression, which outlast the pollen season. Similarly ACTH gel
and depot tetrasocatrin have been found useful in relieving hay fever,[43,44]
and perennial rhinitis.[45] However, the need for frequent injections and occasional development of allergic reactions makes their use in children of
limited value.

Although intra-nasal use of corticosteroids has been tried during the
last twenty years, the frequent incidence of serious side-effects has not
justified their general use[46] until recently. The development of
beclomethasone dipropionate and dexamethasone valerate aerosols which
possess high topical activity compared with a relative absence of systemic
effects now make their use possible.[47] The treatment must be given two

to four times daily and the relief of symptoms usually occurs after a period of days. Between 60 and 80 per cent of individuals with seasonal allergic rhinitis will derive benefit from intranasal beclomethasone dipropionate or betamethasone valerate.[14,49,50]

Similar results have been obtained in subjects prone to perennial rhinitis although few studies have so far been published on that subject in children.[51-53] The beneficial response is obtained usually within a week, but in the occasional child, improvement may not occur for a number of weeks. Side effects such as adrenal cortical suppression have not been described. Nasal infection with *Candida albicans* is infrequent although in some patients organisms can be grown from mouth washings.[52]

Table 6.2 Intranasal corticosteroids in rhinitis

Reference	Year	Type of rhinitis	No. of patients	% improvement	Remarks
54	1974	Seasonal	72	78	—
49	1975	Seasonal	26	77	Betamethasone valerate
50	1975	Seasonal	18	95	Children only. Beclomethasone diproprionate. Need for antihistamines reduced
51	1974	Perennial	25	75	—
52	1976	Perennial	30	73	Comparison with antihistamine (Actifed)
53	1977	Perennial	27	65	Improvement seen within 5 days. Peak expiratory flow rates were measured through the nose to detect the degree of nasal obstruction

e. *Sodium cromoglycate BP and intranasal steroids.* Comparison of intranasal sodium cromoglycate BP and beclomethasone dipropionate in 20 subjects with seasonal rhinitis showed significant reduction of symptoms scores (eye and nasal irritation, nasal discharge and obstruction, sneezing) but no differences between the two treatments.[55] In another study[56] of 40 patients with seasonal rhinitis, administration of 400 μg/day of intranasal bethamethasone valerate was of greater benefit in relieving symptoms than 80 mg/day of sodium cromoglycate ($P < 0.01$).

f. *Immunotherapy.* Noon[57] in 18 patients with hay fever, showed that administration of injections of boiled timothy grass pollen extracts over a period of time reduced symptoms during the following season in a majority of his patients. Although numerous studies have been published since then, controversy still exists regarding the efficacy of this mode of treatment, especially if it is remembered that 35 per cent of subjects with seasonal rhinitis improve following a course of placebo.[58] Undoubtedly the results depend on the type and composition of extract used, the frequency of dosages and duration of treatment, as well as atmospheric concentrations of allergens and the possibility that symptoms might have arisen following exposure to different allergens.[59-61]

Methods

Immunotherapy with allergen extracts consisted initially of a series of injections of watery extracts of allergens (the water being emulsified) in oil so that the allergens slowly diffused into the tissues (repository method) from the injection site. These methods, however, were associated with unpleasant side-effects such as exacerbation of rhinitis, asthma, anaphylaxis and local or general tissue swelling and pain. The use of alum-precipitated pollen extracts has allowed fewer injections but not uncommonly causes more local reactions. The alum-precipitated pyridine extracts cause fewer systemic and local reactions than the aqueous extracts.[62-65] Since the number of injections is also reduced, this type of treatment clearly has advantages in children. Other types of extracts are allergoids which are formed when pollen extracts are treated with formaldehyde in order to reduce reactions but induce formation of blocking antibody,[66] and amino-acid (tyrosine) adsorbed extracts which allow slow release of allergens from an injection site because of precipitating properties in the presence of allergens. Tyrosine itself is fully metabolised by the body.[67-71]

Mechanism of immunotherapy

The object of hypsensitisation is to stimulate the production of specific IgG blocking antibodies which although reacting with allergens do not lead to mast cell sensitivity and release of chemical mediators, and to avoid or reduce the production of specific IgE antibodies. Undoubtedly other immunological changes occur following hyposensitisation, e.g. decreased lymphocyte transformation, decrease of T cell response, decreased histamine release from basophils, etc. which may be responsible for the clinical improvement. Although many studies have demonstrated significant rises of specific IgG levels following a course of treatment (usually within three months) subsequent exposure to or challenge with the allergens has not prevented an appreciable increase of specific IgE levels. Moreover, although one can demonstrate immunological changes these may not correlate well with exacerbations of symptoms. In general, the skin sensitivity tests are not altered by even prolonged courses of immunotherapy.[59,64,69,71-78]

Indications

A child who shows a Type I hypersensitivity reaction to inhalant allergens such as grass pollens or the house dust mite and who has not improved significantly following adequate trials with intranasal sodium cromoglycate or steroid aerosols should be considered for hyposensitisation. In general because of the risks of possible generalised reactions immunotherapy should not be employed in children under the age of 6 years.

Four seasonal allergic rhinitis injections must be given pre-seasonally. If treatment is not effective the injections are repeated again before the subsequent two seasons. It is important that the doctor administers the injections himself and keeps the child under observation for at least 30 minutes afterwards. Adrenaline and hydrocortisone acetate should always be available when hyposensitisation is carried out. Local reactions are rarely troublesome and respond to antihistamine agents. Generalised reactions such as urticaria or bronchospasm respond quickly to adrenaline BP 1:1000 solution 0·2–0·5 ml s.c. The injection should be given adjacent to the hyposensitisation injection site. For the most severe reactions hydrocortisone acetate 200 mg should be given i.v. immediately.

Composition and dosages of allergen extracts

1. *Allpyral G* and *Alavac-P.* (pyridine alum-precipitated allergens in aqueous soln. of 0·9% saline and using 0·4% phenol as preservative).

Extracts of pollens of five grasses (Cocksfoot, meadow fescue, perennial rye, timothy and Yorkshire fog).

Extracts are standardised on protein nitrogen unit basis

2. *Allpyral Specific.*

a. Containing various flower mixture
b. Tree and mould pollens
c. *D. pteronyssinus* and mite fortified house dust
d. Feather mixture
e. Stinging insect extracts of bee and wasp venoms.

Available in three types of sets:

(1) Initial treatment set:

(a) Vial No. 1 (green label) contains extract of 100 PNU/ml strength;

(b) Vial No. 2 (blue label) contains extract of 1000 PNU/ml strength;

(c) Vial No. 3 (black label) contains extract of 10,000 PNU/ml strength.

(2) Maintenance treatment sets:
Composition as in (c) above.

(3) Special sets:
These consist of vials (black label) of 10 PNU/ml strength.

Allpyral *D. pteronyssinus* consists of three vials of 100, 1000 and 4000 PNU/ml strength extracts.

Dose and course of treatment

(a) *Seasonal rhinitis.* Pre-seasonal course of 8–10 s.c. injections given every four weeks. The course to finish three to four weeks before pollination. In some young children it is best to start initially with 10 PNU/ml extract strength and gradually increase. The course should be repeated for three seasons.

(b) *Perennial rhinitis.* The course should be as for seasonal rhinitis but maintenance treatment may be required for a considerable period of time. If employed injections should be given every four weeks.

3. *Pollinex* (glutaraldehyde modified extracts adsorbed to tyrosine) — Extract from 12 varieties of grasses (bent, brome, cocksfoot, crested dogstail, false oat, fescue, meadow foxtail, meadow grass, rye grass, timothy, vernal and Yorkshire fog). Phenol used as a preservative.

Initial treatment:

(a) Vial 1   300 Noon Units.
(b) Vial 2   800 Noon Units.
(c) Vial 3   2000 Noon Units.

Injections are given every 7 or 14 days and should always be completed by early May. Maintenance courses should be given for the next three seasons.

4. *Migen* (glutaraldehyde *D. pteronyssinus* extract adsorbed to tyrosine)
   Each course consists of 6 vials of 4, 10, 25, 60, 150 and 400 Noon Units respectively. Injections are given s.c. every 7 to 14 days. Maintenance therapy remains empirical.

5. *SDV* (specific desensitising vaccine)
   Aqueous formulation of three 10 ml multidose vials of allergens in graded strengths. Each vaccine is prepared according to clinical data and tests. As a rule vials contain extracts of eight allergen mixtures.

    (a) Green label vial $\frac{1}{64}$ strength
    (b) Buff label vial $\frac{1}{64}$ strength

    (c) Red label vial $\frac{1}{8}$ strength

Dosage:
   Three courses of six injections each of 0·1 ml, 0·2 ml, 0·3 ml, 0·5 ml, 0·7 ml and 1 ml. For younger children further dilutions can be made. Maintenance treatment can be used by repeating injections weekly or monthly or 1 ml from the red label vial for 6 to 18 injections.

Benefits of immunotherapy

Significant improvement is obtained in seasonal allergic rhinitis. Overall between 70 and 80 per cent of children will benefit from a course of treatment for the subsequent two or three seasons. The results in perennial rhinitis are less clear. There is evidence that subjects who show most benefit are those who have had prolonged courses of immunotherapy and at times the relief of symptoms may occur only after prolonged use, e.g. up to two years. After treatment is discontinued some children remain well but others relapse within a few weeks or months and may improve again if hyposensitisation is restarted. The most evidence has accumulated in hyposensitisation with *D. pteronyssinus* extract. It is a common and important allergen causing rhinitis and asthma in children.[80] Table summarises some of the results obtained in allergic rhinitis.

g. *Nasal desensitisation.* In this method the allergen in aqueous solution is sprayed in the nose.[26,85,87] Initially very dilute solutions are used in order to produce minimal symptoms. A course consists of 10 to 12 doses given every few days. A double blind trial of 42 children with pollenosis demonstrated 70 per cent improvement in clinical state and nasal FEV.[86] Similar findings have been repeated in adults.[85] Although no serious side-effects have been reported, in another study it was shown that

Table 6.3   Effects of hyposensitisation in allergic rhinitis

Reference	Year	Type of rhinitis	No. of patients	% improve-ment	Remarks
81	1954	Seasonal	198	79	Placebo study. 33% placebo subjects improved
82	1968	Seasonal	26	77	Placebo study. 8% placebo subjects improved
83	1976	Seasonal	100	73	Not controlled. Tyrosine adsorbed vaccine used. 16% had local reactions
84	1975	Seasonal	22	55* 18** 23***	Children only
79	1973	Perennial	91	64	But 66% of controls also improved
65	1976	Perennial	52	85	—
71	1977	Perennial	66	75	Placebo controlled. Course consisted of 18–22 weekly injections

*—Complete relief; **—good response; ***—slight response.

proteinuria and systemic symptoms could be reproduced by repeated nasal exposure to the allergens during hyposensitisation.[88]

h. *Surgical procedures.* The value of palliative operations is largely speculative and undetermined. Removal of nasal polyps has received most attention. However, cryotherapy, at times successful when vasomotor symptoms predominate, may be effective in perennial rhinitis especially when nasal obstruction and excessive mucus secretion is present. In one study of 288 patients, relief of symptoms was obtained in 76 per cent during a 4 year observation period.[89]

i. *Newer anti-allergic drugs.* Recently a number of preliminary studies has been described of potent agents, whose mode of action is similar to sodium cromoglycate. In one study of 10 patients with allergic rhinitis a phenanthroline agent administered as an aerosol prior to exposure was associated with a high degree of protection following allergen challenge, and in a clinical trial of 24 patients with seasonal rhinitis, 50 per cent showed significant improvement during the pollen season.[90-95]

Nasal polyps (coined by Galen after sea polyp)

These are hyperplastic and oedematous swellings arising on the lateral aspects of the nasal cavity, and which derive from either the middle turbinates, or from herniations of the mucosa (ostia) of the ethmoid or maxillary sinuses. The polyp becomes congested due to venous stasis caused by venous constriction, gravity and antigen antibody reactions within the mucosa. The polyps are covered by columnar ciliated epithelium which may be absent in the presence of chronic infection. Some blood vessels, mucous glands, plasma cells, lymphocytes and eosinophils are often seen.[96,104]

Clinically the polyps vary in number and size, have the appearance of an 'oyster' or 'grapes', i.e. smooth, solid, grey and glistening and mobile to touch. During exacerbations of rhinitis polyps look inflamed, presenting a reddish appearance. The majority of children with polyps become mouth breathers and develop nocturnal coughs due to the post-nasal mucous discharge. Although stated to be rare in children[97] they were found in 8 per cent of 86 asthmatics, 5 per cent of 23 children with vasomotor rhinitis and 4 per cent of children with cystic fibrosis.[98] Indeed, cystic fibrosis should be excluded first.[102] Review of the literature reveals that polyps are often present in subjects with asthma (23 to 42 per cent) but the incidence of asthma in subjects with nasal polyps ranges from 2·9 to 72 per cent. However, in a review of 1298 asthmatic children, nasal polyps were found only in those who were also sensitive to aspirin (27 per cent of 15 children).[97] Similar findings were recorded in a study of 3000 allergic adults.[100]

The immunological mechanisms involved are uncertain although the release of histamine, slow-reacting substance, eosinophil chemotactic factor of anaphylaxis,[105] activation of the complement system, kinins and inhibition of prostaglandin synthesis have been judged to be of importance.[99,103]

In general aspirin sensitivity appears to arise only after the polyps have occurred.[101]

The treatment consists of removal of the polyps often requiring repeated procedures or prolonged courses of intranasal steroids or ACTH which have been found of particular value in children.

Indications for the removal of adenoids and tonsils in the allergic child

There is evidence that tonsillar and adenoidal tissues contain immunoglobulins such as IgA, IgG and IgM. Following adenotonsillectomy the release of such antibodies in to the nasopharynx is reduced.[106,111] Also a significant number of children with upper respiratory tract infections due to *Haemophilus influenzae* were found to have low serum levels of IgA and still continued to have frequent recurrences after the operation.[107] The controversy regarding long-term benefits of adenotonsillectomy remains unsettled.[108–110]

Chronic enlargement of adenoids and tonsils is a common clinical finding in children with untreated allergic rhinitis. However, such hypertrophy subsides following treatment of the rhinitis. The removal of tonsils or adenoids in untreated allergic children is followed by re-growth of these tissues. Surgery should be considered in those children who get recurrent attacks of acute tonsillitis associated with otitis media, chronic Eustachian tube obstruction (glue ear) and conductive deafness, have normal serum IgA levels and possibly those with chronic streptococcal sore-throats and a family history of rheumatic fever. Above all, before the removal of large tonsils and adenoids is considered, allergy should be excluded first, because without doubt conservative management will be of greater and more lasting value than elective surgery.

References

1. Negus, V. (1954) The function of the paranasal sinuses. *Acta Otolaryngol,* **44,** 408.
2. Protez, A. W. (1953) Respiratory air currents and their clinical aspects, Semon Lecture. *J. Laryng.,* **67,** 11.
3. Korkis, F. B. (1958) The functions of the nose. In: *Recent Advances in Otolaryngology.* 3rd ed., p. 206. London: Churchill.
4. Holzel, A. (1968) The allergic toddler. *The Practitioner,* **200,** 369.
5. Hagy, H. W. and Settipane, G. A. (1975) Risks of developing asthma and allergic rhinitis: a 7 year follow up study of 903 college students. *J. Allergy Clin. Immunol.,* **55,** 124.
6. Perkin, J. N. (1972) Allergy in general practice. *The Practitioner,* **208,** 776.
7. Carr, R. D., Berke, M. and Becker, W. S. (1964) Incidence of atopy in the general population. *Archs Dermatol.,* **89,** 27.
8. Blair, H. (1974) The incidence of asthma, hay fever and infantile eczema in an East End London group practice of 9145 patients. *Clin. Allergy,* **4,** 389.
9. Viner, A. S. and Jackman, N. (1976) Retrospective survey of 1271 patients diagnosed as perennial rhinitis. *Clin. Allergy,* **6,** 251.
10. Dolovich, J., Back, N. and Arbesman, C. E. (1970) Kinin-like activity in nasal secretions of allergic patients. *Int. archs Allergol.,* **38,** 337.
11. Bryant, D. H., Turnbull, L. W. and Kay, A. B. (1977) Eosinophil chemotaxis to an ECP–A tetrapeptide and histamine: the response in various disease states. *Clin. Allergy,* **7,** 219.
12. Watanabe, K., Hasegawa, M., Saito, Y. and Takayama, S. (1977) Eosinophilic leucocytes in nasal allergy—movement of enzymes. *Clin. Allergy,* **7,** 263.
13. Kaliner, M., Wasserman, S. I. and Austen, K. F. (1973) Immunologic release of chemical mediators from human nasal polyps. *New Eng. Med. J.,* **289,** 277.
14. Mygind, N. (1973) Local effect of intranasal beclomethasone dipropionate aerosol in hay fever. *Br. med. J.,* **IV,** 464.

15. Connell, J. T. (1969) Quantitative intranasal pollen challenges. The priming effect in allergic rhinitis. *J. Allergy*, **43**, 33.
16. Mygind, N., Viner, A. S. and Jackman, N. (1974) Histology of nasal mucosa in normals and in patients with perennial rhinitis. *Rhinology*, **XII**, 131.
17. Murray, A. B. (1970) Nasal secretion eosinophilia in children with allergic rhinitis. *Ann. Allergy*, **28**, 142.
18. Taylor, G. and Shivalkar, P. R. (1971) 'Arthus-type' reactivity in the nasal airways and skin in pollen sensitive subjects. *Clin. Allergy*, **1**, 407.
19. Solomon, W. R. (1966) Comparative effects of transient body surface cooling, recumbency and induced obstruction in allergic rhinitis and control subjects. *J. Allergology*, **37**, 216.
20. Murray, A. B. (1972) Appearance of the turbinates and nasal allergy in children. *Annls Allergy*, **30**, 245.
21. Lowell, F. C. (1967) Clinical aspects of eosinophilia in atopic disease. *J. Am. med. Ass.*, **202**, 875.
22. Whitcomb, N. J. (1965) Allergy therapy in serous otitis media associated with allergic rhinitis. *Annls Allergy*, **23**, 232.
23. Stewart, J. P. and Kawa, M. Z. (1954) Histological changes in allergic rhinitis. *J. Laryngol.*, **68**, 193.
24. Ahlstedt, S., Eriksson, N., Lindgren, S. and Roth, A. (1974) Specific IgE determination by RAST compared with skin and provocation tests in allergy diagnosis with birch, timothy pollen and dog epithelium allergens. *Clin. Allergy*, **4**, 131.
25. Deuschl, H. and Johansson, S. G. O. (1977) Specific IgE antibodies in nasal secretion from patients with allergic rhinitis and with negative or weakly positive RAST on the serum. *Clin. Allergy*, **7**, 195.
26. Taylor, G. and Shivalkar, P. R. (1971) Changes in nasal airways resistance on antigenic challenge in allergic rhinitis. *Clin. Allergy*, **1**, 63.
27. Kuzemko, J. A. (1978) unpublished observations.
28. Penaud, A., Nourrit, J., Timon-David, P. and Charpin, J. (1977) Results of a controlled trial of the acaride Paragerm on *Dermatophagoides* spp. in dwelling houses. *Clin. Allergy*, **7**, 49.
29. Capel, L. H. and McKelvie, P. (1971) Disodium cromoglycate in hay fever. *Lancet*, **I**, 575.
30. Holopainen, E., Backman, A. and Salo, O. P. (1971) Effect of DSCG on seasonal allergic rhinitis. *Lancet*, **I**, 55.
31. Engström, I. (1971) The effect of disodium cromoglycate on nasal provocation tests in children with seasonal allergic rhinitis. *Acta allerg.*, **26**, 101.
32. Thorne, M. G. and Bradeer, W. H. (1972) Disodium cromoglycate in the treatment of perennial allergic rhinitis. *Acta allerg.*, **27**, 307.
33. Girard, J. P. and Bertrand, J. (1975) Study of a 2% solution of sodium cromoglycate in perennial rhinitis assessed by subjective and objective parameters. *Clin. Allergy*, **5**, 301.
34. Frostad, A. B. (1977) The treatment of seasonal allergic rhinitis with a 2% aqueous solution of sodium cromoglycate delivered by a metered dose nasal spray. *Clin. Allergy*, **7**, 347.
35. Taylor, G. and Shivalkar, P. R. (1971) Disodium cromoglycate: laboratory studies and clinical trial in allergic rhinitis. *Clin. Allergy*, **2**, 189.
36. Blair, H. and Viner, S. A. (1975) A double blind trial of a 2% solution of sodium cromoglycate in perennial rhinitis. *Clin. Allergy*, **5**, 139.
37. König, P. and Godfrey, S. (1973) Prevalence of exercise-induced bronchial lability in families of children with asthma. *Archs dis. Child*, **48**, 513.
38. Parker, C. D., Bilbo, R. E. and Reed, C. E. (1965) Methacholine aerosol as test for bronchial asthma. *Ann. inter. Med.*, **115**, 452.
39. McNichol, K. N. and Williams, H. E. (1973) Spectrum of asthma in children—II. Allergic components. *Br. med. J.*, **IV**, 12.
40. Godfrey, R. C. and Griffiths, M. (1976) The prevalence of immediate positive tests

to *Dermatophagoides pteronyssinus* and grass pollen in school children. *Clin. Allergy*, **6,** 79.

41. Ganderton, M. A. and James, V. H. T. (1970) Clinical and endocrine side-effects of methylprednisolone acetate as used in hay fever. *Br. med. J.*, **I,** 267.

42. Melotte G. (1973) Depot corticosteroid preparations in hay fever. *The Practitioner*, **210,** 282.

43. Parr, E. J. (1976) Hay fever treated with ACTH gel. *Clin. Allergy*, **6,** 479.

44. McAllen, M. (1972) The prevention and treatment of hay fever. *The Practitioner*, **208,** 757.

45. Nelson, J. K., Mackay, J. S., Sheridan B. and Weaver, J. A. (1966) Intermittent therapy with corticotrophin. *Lancet*, **II,** 78.

46. Bagratuni, L. (1960) A comparative study of topical steroids, antihistamines and pollen vaccine in the treatment of hay fever and hay asthma. *Annls Allergy*, **18,** 859.

47. Wilson, L. (1974) The dissociation of topical from systemic effect in corticosteroids. *Postgrad. Med. J.*, **4,** 50, Suppl. 7.

48. Morrison-Smith, J. (1971) Disodium cromoglycate in hay fever. *Lancet*, **I,** 295.

49. Archer, G. J., Thomas, A. K. and Harding, S. M. (1975) Intranasal betamethasone valerate in the treatment of seasonal rhinitis. *Clin. Allergy*, **5,** 285.

50. Prahl, P., Wilken-Jensen, K. and Mygind, N. (1975) Beclomethasone dipropionate aerosol in treatment of hay fever in children. *Archs dis. Child.*, **50,** 875.

51. Gibson, G. J., Maberly, D. J., Lal, S., Ali, M. M. and Butler, A. G. (1974) Double-blind cross-over trial comparing intranasal beclomethasone dipropionate and placebo in perennial rhinitis. *Brit. med. J.*, **IV,** 503.

52. Harding, S. M. and Heath, S. (1976) Intranasal steroid aerosol in perennial rhinitis; comparison on antihistamine compound. *Clin. Allergy*, **4,** 291.

53. Lahdensuo, A. and Haahtela, T. (1977) Efficacy of intranasal beclomethasone dipropionate in patients with perennial rhinitis and asthma. *Clin. Allergy*, **7,** 255.

54. Brown, M. H. and Storey, G. (1974) Beclomethasone dipropionate aerosol in the treatment of seasonal asthma and hay fever. *Clin. Allergy*, **4,** 331.

55. Chatterjee, S. S., Nassar, W. Y., Wilson, O. and Butler, A. G. (1974) Intranasal beclomethasone diproprionate and intranasal sodium cromoglycate: a comparative trial. *Clin. Allergy*, **4,** 343.

56. Frankland, A. W. and Walker, S. R. (1975) A comparison of intranasal betamethasone valerate and sodium cromoglycate in seasonal allergic rhinitis. *Clin. Allergy*, **5,** 295.

57. Noon, L. (1911) Prophylactic inoculation for hay fever. *Lancet*, **I,** 1572.

58. Shure, N. (1965) The placebo in allergy. *Annls Allergy*, **23,** 368.

59. Davies, R. R. and Smith, L. P. (1973) Weather and the grass pollen content of the air. *Clin. Allergy*, **4,** 95.

60. Davies, R. R. (1969) Climate and topography in relation to aero-allergens at Davos and London. *Acta allerg.*, **24,** 396.

61. Baldo, B. A. and Uhlenbruck, G. (1977) Allergen standardisation using lectins. *Lancet*, **I,** 802.

62. Frankland, A. W. and Noelpp, B. (1966) Summer hay fever treated with aqueous and alum-precipitated pyridine extracts. *The Practitioner*, **196,** 766.

63. Munro-Ashman, D. (1966) An alum-precipitated pyridine extract in the treatment of hay fever. *The Practitioner*, **196,** 771.

64. Fagerberg, E., Nilzen, A. and Wiholm, S. (1972) Studies in hyposensitisation with Allpyral. *Acta allerg.*, **27,** 1.

65. Munro-Ashman, D. and Frankland, A. W. (1976) Treatment of allergy to house dust with pyridine-extracted alum-precipitated extracts of the house dust mite. *Annls Allergy*, **36,** 95.

66. Norman, P. S., Lichtenstein, L. M. and Winkelwerder, W. L. (1972) Immunotherapy of grass pollen hay fever with grass pollen allergoid. *J. Allergy Clin. Immunol.*, **49,** 114.

67. Johansson, S. G. O., Miller, A. C. M. L., Mullan, N., Overell, B. G., Tees, E. C. and Wheeler, A. (1974) Glutaraldehyde-pollen-tyrosine: Clinical and immunological studies. *Clin. Allergy*, **4**, 255.
68. Miller, A. C. and Tees, E. C. (1974) A metabolizable adjuvant: clinical trial of grass pollen-tyrosine adsorbate. *Clin. Allergy*, **4**, 49.
69. Foucard, T. and Johansson, S. G. O. (1976) Immunological studies *in vitro* and *in vivo* of children with pollenosis given immunotherapy with an aqueous and a glutaraldehyde-treated tyrosine-adsorbed grass pollen extract. *Clin. Allergy*, **6**, 429.
70. Symington, I. S., O'Neill, D. and Kerr, J. W. (1977) Comparison of a glutaraldehyde-modified pollen-tyrosine adsorbate with an alum-precipitated pollen vaccine in the treatment of hay fever. *Clin. Allergy*, **7**, 189.
71. Gabriel, M., Ng, H. K., Allan, W. G. L., Hill, L. E. and Nunn, A. J. (1977) Study of prolonged hyposensitisation with *D. pteronyssinus* extract in allergic rhinitis. *Clin. Allergy*, **7**, 325.
72. Ishizaka, K., Kishimoto, T. and Delespesse, G. (1973) IgE and IgG antibody responses during immunotherapy. *J. Allergy Clin. Immunol.*, **51**, 79.
73. Reisman, R. E., Wypych, J. I. and Arbesman, C. E. (1975) Relationship of immunotherapy, seasonal pollen exposure and clinical response to serum concentrations of total IgE and ragweed-specific IgE. *Int. Archs. Allergy appl. Immunol.*, **48**, 721.
74. Levy, D. A., Lichtenstein, L. M., Goldstein, E. and Ishizaka, K. (1971) Immunologic and cellular changes accompanying the therapy of pollen allergy. *J. clin. Invest.*, **50**, 360.
75. Sadan, N., Rhyne, M. B., Mellits, E. D., Goldstein, E. D., Levy, D. A. and Lichtenstein, L. M. (1969) Immunotherapy of pollenosis in children. Investigation of the immunologic basis of clinical improvement. *New Eng. Med. J.*, **280**, 623.
76. Yunginger, J. W. and Gleich, G. J. (1973) Seasonal changes in IgE antibodies and their relationship to IgG antibodies during immunotherapy for ragweed hay fever. *J. clin. Invest.*, **52**, 1268.
77. Yunginger, J. W. and Gleich, G. J. (1975) The impact of the discovery of IgE on the practice of allergy. *Pediatr. Clin. N. Am.*, **22**, 3.
78. Assem, E. S. and McAllen, M. K. (1973) Changes in challenge tests following hyposensitisation, with mite extract. *Clin. Allergy*, **3**, 161.
79. D'Souza, M. F., Pepys, J., Wells, D., Tai, E., Palmer, F., Overell, B. G., McGrath, I. T. and Megson, M. (1973) Hyposensitisation with *Dermatophagoides pteronyssinus* in house dust allergy: a controlled study of clinical and immunological effects. *Clin. Allergy*, **3**, 177.
80. Kuzemko, J. A. (1976) *Asthma in Children*, p. 5. Tunbridge Wells, Pitman Medical.
81. Frankland, A. W. and Augustin, R. (1954) Prophylaxis of summer hay-fever and asthma. *Lancet*, **I**, 1055.
82. Norman, P. S., Winkelwerder, W. L. and Lichtenstein, L. M. (1968) Immunotherapy of hay fever with ragweed antigen E: comparisons with whole pollen extract and placebos. *J. Allergy*, **42**, 93.
83. Miller, A. C. M. L. (1976) A trial of hyposensitisation in 1974/5 in the treatment of hay fever using gluteraldehyde–pollen–tyrosine adsorbate. *Clin. Allergy*, **6**, 557.
84. Blair, H., Ezeoke, A. and Hobbs, J. R. (1975) IgE, IgG and patient-self tests during slow hyposensitisation to grass pollen. *Clin. Allergy*, **3**, 263.
85. Taylor, G. and Shivalkar, P. R. (1972) Local nasal densitisation in allergic rhinitis. *Clin. Allergy*, **2**, 125.
86. Mehta, S. B. and Morrison Smith, J. (1975) Nasal hyposensitisation and hay fever. *Clin. Allergy*, **5**, 279.
87. Cooke, N. (1974) Pre-seasonal local nasal desensitisation in hay fever. *J. Laryngol. Otol.*, **88**, 1169.
88. Freed, D. L. J. and Taylor, G. (1976) Local nasal desensitisation provoking systemic illness with proteinuria. *Clin. Allergy*, **6**, 173.
89. Puhakka, H. and Rantanen, T. (1977) Cryotherapy as a method of treatment in

allergic and vasomotor rhinitis. *J. Laryng. Otol.*, **91**, 535.

90. Batchelor, J. F., Garland, L. G., Green, A. F., Hughes, D. T. D., Follenfant, M. J., Gorvin, J. H., Hodson, H. F. and Tateson, J. E. (1975) Doxantrazole, an antiallergic agent orally effective in man. *Lancet*, **I**, 1169.

91. Micallef, R. E. and Fenech, F. F. (1977) FPL 57787: A new oral chromogen in the treatment of bronchial asthma. *Allergolog. Immunopathol.*, **5**, 519.

92. Lenney, W., Milner, A. D. and Tyler, R. M. (1977) Comparison of disodium cromoglycate and BRL 10833 activity in blocking exercise induced bronchospasm in asthmatic children. *Allergolog. Immunopathol.*, **5**, 519.

93. Cairns, H. (1977) The development of an orally effective anti-allergic Chromone FPL 57787. *Allergolog. Immunopathol.*, **5**, 520.

94. Vilsvik, J. S. and Jenssen, A. O. (1976) The effect of a new anti-allergic drug ICI 74917, given by aerosol, on nasal stenosis induced allergen. *Clin. Allergy*, **6**, 487.

95. Blair, H. (1977) A trial of ICI 74917 in seasonal allergic rhinitis. *Clin. Allergy*, **4**, 397.

96. Korkis, F. B. (1958) *Recent Advances in Oto-laryngology.* 3rd ed., p. 227. London: Churchill.

97. Falliers, C. J. (1973) Aspirin and subtypes of asthma risk, factor analysis. *J. Allergy Clin. Immunol.*, **52**, 141.

98. Kuzemko, J. A. (1978) Unpublished data.

99. Moloney, J. R. and Collins, J. (1977) Nasal polyps and bronchial asthma. Review article. *Br. J. dis. Chest*, **71**, 1.

100. Caplin, I., Haynes, J. T. and Spahn, J. (1971) Are nasal polyps an allergic phenomenon? *Annls Allergy*, **29**, 631.

101. Wilson, J. A. (1976) Nasal polypi. *Clin. Otolaryngol.*, **1**, 4.

102. Schwachman, H., Kulczycki, L. L. and Mueller, H. L. (1962) Nasal polyposis in patients with cystic fibrosis. *Pediatrics*, **30**, 389.

103. Szczeklik, A., Gryglewski, R. J. and Czerniawska-Mysik, G. (1975) Relationship of inhibition of prostaglandin biosynthesis by analgesics to asthma attacks in aspirin sensitive patients. *Br. med. J.*, **1**, 67.

104. Whiteside, T. L., Rabin, B. S., Zetterberg, O. —. and Criep, L. (1975) The presence of IgE on the surface of lymphocytes in nasal polyps. *J. Allergy Clin. Immunol.*, **55**, 186.

105. Samter, M. and Beers, R. F. (1968) Intolerance to aspirin. Clinical studies and consideration of its pathogenesis. *Annls int. Med.*, **68**, 975.

106. Ogra, P. L. (1971) Effect of tonsillectomy and adenoidectomy on nasapharyngeal antibody response to poliovirus. *New Eng. Med. J.*, **284**, 59.

107. Donovan, R. and Soothill, J. F. (1973) Immunological studies in children undergoing tonsillectomy. *Clin. exp. Immunol.*, **14**, 347.

108. Mawson, S. R., Adlington, R. and Evans, M. (1967) A controlled study evaluation of adeno-tonsillectomy in children. *J. Laryng. Otol.*, **81**, 777.

109. Donovan, R. (1973) Clinical and immunological studies on children undergoing tonsillectomy for repeated sore throats. *Proc. R. Soc. Med.*, **66**, 413.

110. Wood, B., Wong, Y. K. and Theodoridis, C. G. (1972) Paediatricians look at children awaiting adenotonsillectomy. *Lancet*, **II**, 645.

111. Kjellman, N. I. M., Synnerstad, B. and Hansson, L. O. (1976) Atopic allergy and immunoglobulins in children with adenoids and recurrent otitis media. *Acta paediatr. Scand.*, **65**, 593.

CHAPTER 7

Ears

ALLERGIC REACTIONS MAY affect the external, middle and inner ears.

External ear contact dermatitis

The evidence of hypersensitivity is usually obvious. A history of contact is always present. In young babies it may be due to certain soaps or contact with animal epithelium and in older children as reaction to metals such as earrings and cosmetics. Contact dermatitis behind the ear is often due to the frames of spectacles or occasionally hair sprays, while dermatitis of the external auditory meatus is almost always caused by a prolonged use of ear drops.

Clinical examination will show erythematous rash with a tendency to vesicle formation. Since there is associated itching, secondary infection is not uncommonly present and causes crusting and oozing of the lesions.

Management is straightforward and includes the avoidance of precipitating factors, local application of a dilute corticosteroid ointment for two to three days only and occasionally, if pruritus is troublesome, oral administration of antihistamines for two to three days.

Atopic dermatitis

The external ear may be involved as a part of generalised atopic dermatitis involving other parts of the body. The clinical features and management are as has been previously described on pages 43–52. In the young baby it should be distinguished from seborrhoeic dermatitis (see page 44).

Middle ear–serous otitis media

In this condition there appears a sterile effusion in the middle ear. It may occur suddenly giving rise to acute symptoms or over a period of time as part of an upper respiratory tract disease. Indeed, it not uncommonly presents as a case of deafness. The accumulation of fluid is due to the failure of air replacement in the obstructed Eustachian tube leading to vacuum formation. An effusion occurs because the pressure surrounding the blood vessels of the mucosa of the vacuum is decreased. There is some evidence that with recurrent attacks squamous metaplasia may occur and an increase in the plasma cells, lymphocytes and goblet cells and possibly some dysfunction of the Eustachian tube itself.[1,2] The effusing fluid as obtained by aspiration (myringotomy) looks thin suggesting a transudate but occasionally is thick especially in the presence of an infection.

Results of analysis of the effusion fluid have been conflicting. Some studies have demonstrated an increased amount of IgE and eosinophils.[3-6] That immunological reactions can occur in the ear has been shown by demonstrating hypersensitivity in the guinea pig by challenging an ear immunised by bovine serum albumin.[7] The studies of the effects of vacuum on the tympanic cavity have demonstrated that obstruction to the nasopharynx and Eustachian tube can result in fluid accumulation within the middle ear.[8,9]

Many factors have been implicated in causation of serous otitis media in children. Various aetiological factors have been suggested such as the respiratory syncytial virus, chronic hypertrophy of the tonsils and adenoids, chronic sinusitis, dental malocclusion, congenital abnormalities of the Eustachian tube, disturbance of muscle function, trauma, hypothyroidism and allergy.[10-16]

Allergic serous otitis media

A positive history of atopy in the child is present in between 11 and 70 per cent of children and positive family history in 48 per cent of the children.[16-19] The most common allergens involved are foods such as eggs, chicken, chocolate, corn and wheat,[1] and inhalants as house dust and grass pollens. In some studies improvement followed elimination of the offending allergen and relapse on its introduction.[14] In animal studies, serous effusion with raised eosinophil count and protein were produced on oral challenge with cow's milk, horse serum, etc.[7,20,21,23]

The onset of symptoms is usually between the ages of 2 and 6 in at least 90 per cent of children. The highest incidence occurs during the winter months and early spring. Boys are twice as likely to be affected as girls. In one study,[22] 20 per cent of five-year-old children entering school were found to have fluid-filled middle ears. The surgical treatment of this condition accounts for 60 per cent of surgery in children under the age of 10 years in an ENT unit.[23]

Diagnosis

Symptoms are often vague and some degree of deafness may be the only presenting feature which is commented on by parents or teachers. Some children complain of recurrent earache, buzzing sensation in the ear on changing of posture or being 'blocked up'. An older child may complain of his voice sounding like an echo and a tinnitus which is low-pitched.

The examination of the tympanic membrane may show a whitish appearance or bluish-grey discoloration. The classical mirror like reflection is usually absent and landmarks are obscured. The tympanic membrane may be retracted, the drums appear thick, immobile and scarred. It is most unusual to see a classical meniscus fluid level with air bubbles because in the majority of children the effusion fills the middle ear completely.

Any child suspected of serous otitis media should have an immediate audiometric examination which will show conductive hearing loss of between 10 and 50 dB over all the test frequencies. Audiometry may show a certain degree of variability depending on the degree of tubal obstruction and drainage and not uncommonly changes are observed if the audiogram is repeated on a number of occasions.

X-ray examination of the sinuses and mastoids should be done routinely. These may demonstrate definite haziness, which in the allergic child, is usually bilateral and involving ethmoidal and maxiliary sinuses.

The most common complication is superimposed acute suppurative otitis media which may involve the mastoid. Delayed treatment or inadequate treatment of supperative otitis media may lead to adhesions or a permanent impairment of hearing. A cholestatoma may also rarely occur.[24] It is possible that minor speech problems in the very young child may have their origins in the unhealthy middle ear.

For a concise review of allergy and secretory otitis media, the reader is referred to the proceedings of the Symposium on Pediatric Allergy.[30]

Treatment

Prompt advice from an ear, nose and throat surgeon is essential.

If there is evidence of other respiratory tract allergy, the use of nasal vaso-constrictive decongestants for three to four days may be effective or a course of oral antihistamines for four to five days.

In a six week clinical evaluation of three agents (Brompheniramine maleate 4 mg, Phenyleparine hydrochloride 5 mg, and Phenylpropanolamine hydrochloride 5 mg) in 88 children with bilateral secretory otitis media, none produced any significant improvement of symptoms. Interestingly children with otalgia did best and all presenting with deafness required surgical intervention.[23] Antibiotics will be required if bacterial infection is present. The practice of autoinflation four times a day may occasionally be successful in displacing the fluid (mouth closed, one nostril obstructed with finger and forceful blowout with the other nostril—ears should 'pop').

It is likely that the prolonged use of intranasal sodium cromoglycate or one of the steroid aerosols in the management of allergic rhinitis may result in a decreased incidence of secretory otitis media. If there is no appreciable improvement with 10 days, surgical treatment should be considered. It consists of myringotomy, fluid aspiration and often insertion of plastic grommets for ventilation and equalatic pressure. Although hearing is restored immediately about 10 to 15 per cent of children have recurrent episodes and some develop tympanosclerosis. However, the long-term results of this procedure are so far unknown.[25-27] The removal of tonsils and adenoids in such children is of little lasting benefit as regrowth of tissues quickly occur following operation. In the event of flying, a course of decongestants should be used for two to three days.

Inner ear

Although Meniere's disease (disorder affecting cochlea and vestibular apparatus associated with vertigo, tinnitus, recurrent hearing loss and occasionally nystagmus) is rare in children and its pathogenesis undetermined, allergic causes have been occasionally implicated especially food hypersensitivity. Improvement followed efficient treatment of the underlying allergy.[28,29] It is thus important to bear such a possibility in mind in a child presenting with vertigo and tinnitus.

References

1. Hentzer, E. (1972) Ultrastructure of the middle-ear mucosa in secretory otitis media—I. serous effusion. *Acta Otolaryngol.*, **73**, 394, 467.
2. Bernstein, J. M. and Hayes, E. R. (1971) Middle ear mucosa in health and disease. *Archs Otolaryngol.*, **94**, 30.
3. Bauer, F. (1970) Glue ear. *Br. med. J.*, **I**, 111.
4. Ishikawa, T., Bernstein, J. and Reisman, R. E. (1972) Secretory otitis media: Immunologic studies of middle ear secretions. *J. Allergy Clin. Immunol.*, **50**, 319.
5. Lamp, C. B. (1973) Chronic secretory otitis media: immunologic studies of middle ear secretions. *Laryngoscope*, **83**, 276.
6. Philips, M. J., Knight, N. J., Manning, H., Abbot, A. L. and Tripp, W. G. (1974) IgE and secretory otitis media. *Lancet*, **II**, 1176.
7. Hopp, E. S., Elevitch, F. R., Pumphrey, R. E., Irving, T. E. and Hoffman, P. W. (1964) Serous otitis media—an 'immune' therapy. *Laryngoscope*, **74**, 1149.
8. Sadé, J. (1966) Pathology and pathogenesis of serous otitis media. *Archs Otolaryngol.*, **84**, 297.
9. Flisberg, K. (1970) The effects of vacuum on the tympanic cavity. In: *Symposium on Eustachian Tube Problems.* Ed. by Donaldson, J. A., Vol. 3, p. 3. *Otolaryngologic Clinics of N. America.*
10. Berglund, B., Salmivalli, A. and Toivanen, P. (1966) Isolation of respiratory syncytial virus from middle ear exudates of infants. *Acta Otolaryngol.*, **61**, 475.
11. Kapun, Y. P. (1964) Serous otitis media in children. *Archs Otolaryngol.*, **79**, 38.
12. Rapp, D. J. and Fahey, D. J. (1975) Allergy and chronic secretory otitis media. *Pediatr. Clin. N. Am.*, **22**, 259.

13. Miglets, A. (1973) The experimental production of allergic middle ear effusion. *Laryngoscope,* **83,** 1355.

14. Lecks, H. I. (1961) Allergic aspects of serous otitis media in childhood. *N.Y. J. Med.,* **61,** 2737.

15. Senturia, B. H. (1960) Allergic manifestations in otologic disease. *Laryngoscope,* **70,** 287.

16. Kjellman, N. I. M., Synnerstad, B. and Hansson, L. O. (1976) Atopic allergy and immunoglobulins in children with adenoids and recurrent otitis media. *Acta paediatr. Scand.,* **65,** 593.

17. Freeman, M. S. and Freeman, R. J. (1960) Serous otitis media. *Amer. J. Dis. Child.,* **99,** 683.

18. Davison, F. W. (1966) Middle-ear problems in childhood. *J. Am. med. Ass.,* **196,** 834.

19. Dees, S. C. and Lefkowitz, D. (1972) Secretory otitis media in allergic children. *Am. J. Dis. Child.,* **124,** 364.

20. Draper, W. L. (1967) Secretory otitis media in children: A study of 540 children. *Laryngoscope,* **77,** 636.

21. McGovern, J. P., Haywood, T. J. and Fernandez, A. A. (1970) Allergy secretory otitis media: an analysis of 512 cases. *J. Am. med. Ass.,* **200,** 124.

22. Brooks, D. N. (1969) The use of the electro-acoustic impedance bridge in the assessment of middle ear function. *J. inter. Audiol.,* **8,** 563.

23. Fraser, J. G., Mehta, M. and Fraser, P. M. (1972) The medical treatment of secretory otitis media—A clinical trial of three commonly used regimes. *J. of Larynology and Otology,* **9,** 757.

24. Sadé, J. and Haley, A. (1976) The natural history of chronic otitis media. *J. Laryng. Otol.,* **8,** 743.

25. Birrell, J. F. (1976) Otitis media. *Br. med. J.,* **1,** 443.

26. Kärjä, J., Jokinen, K. and Seppälä, A. (1977) Temporal bone findings in the late stage of secretory otitis media. *J. Laryng. Otol.,* **2,** 127.

27. Yagi, H. I. A. (1977) Secretory otitis media in children. The surgical treatment. *J. Laryng. Otol.,* **9,** 267.

28. Schuknecht, H. F. (1968) Correlation of pathology with symptoms of Menier's disease. *Otolaryngol. Clin. N. Am.,* **1,** 433.

29. Clemis, J. D. (1974) Cochleovestibular disorders and allergy. *Otolaryngol. Clin. N. Am.,* **7,** 757.

30. Reisman, R. E. and Bernstein, J. (1975) Allergy and secretory otitis media: Clinical and immunological studies. *Pediatr. Clin. N. Am.,* **22,** 251.

CHAPTER 8

Asthma

THE PATHOGENESIS OF asthma (Greek—breathe hard) remains not fully understood. It must, therefore, be defined in functional and clinical terms:

'It is a condition of altered dynamic state of respiratory passages due to the action of diverse stimuli resulting in airways obstruction of varying degree and duration and reversible partially or completely, spontaneously or under treatment.[1]

Asthma is a familial condition but the environmental component plays a predominant role. Many triggering factors responsible for attacks of asthma are well understood. The discovery of IgE and improved techniques of bronchial provocation testing have added to our understanding of the condition. However, there is still much to be gained by classifying asthmatic children on a clinical basis, i.e. by observing daily changes in peak-flow rates, as these may help greatly in their management.[2]

Incidence

The true incidence of childhood asthma remains unknown. Up to adolescence 2 to 3 per cent of boys have asthma and 1 to 2 per cent of girls. At least half of adults with asthma and hay fever will have developed their first symptoms during childhood. A suggestion has been made that there has been an increase in the incidence of asthma in children during the last few years in England and Wales.

Mortality

The mortality rates vary between 1 and 4 per cent. The number of deaths in England and Wales from asthma per 100,000 children aged 5 to 14 is between 25 and 35 each year, excluding the years 1963–1966 when the number of deaths increased considerably. The reasons for this change in mortality have been fully discussed. Since 1967 the death rate from asthma in the United Kingdom has declined to the pre-1960 years.

Prognosis

The knowledge of factors affecting prognosis is poorly understood. It has been suggested that the age of onset and the relationship to allergy may be important prognostic factors. It has been stated that if asthma starts during the first 2 years of life, outlook for prolonged remission is much worse than if symptoms develop during school years. The presence of another atopic disease such as hay fever or atopic dermatitis implies a poor outlook. Some studies have suggested that early hyposensitisation may lead to a better outlook for the asthmatic child.

A number of long-term observations regarding prognosis of childhood asthma have been published. On average observations have been made between 5 years and 20 years. An analysis of seven studies involving 2294 children showed that 40 per cent became symptom free, 34·5 per cent improved, 24 per cent remained unchanged, 1 per cent deteriorated and 0·5 per cent died.[1]

In a recent study of 267 children followed up for more than 20 years, 52 per cent were almost completely free of symptoms, 21 per cent had one or two episodes of asthma every year and 27 per cent had remissions for at least 3 years—seven children died, three during attacks of asthma.[3] The study suggested that the severity of the initial episode of asthma, artificial feeding, presence of hay fever or eczema and a positive family history of atopy in a first degree relative were associated with poor outlook which was uninfluenced by the age of onset of asthma, the sex of the child or positive skin tests.

Physiology and pathology

The basic abnormality in asthma consists of bronchial muscle constriction and secretion of mucus. The individuals appear to react excessively to stimuli which are without any significant effect in a normal subject. The nature of mechanisms involved is still unknown. The flow of air and normal tone depend on the existence of interaction of the two components of the autonomic nervous system and tissue receptors acting on them. The stimuli are transmitted by various chemical mediators acting on the receptors which are sensitive to them such as the alpha and beta receptors.

Airway resistance is increased and the maximum expiratory flow decreased in children with severe asthma. This suggests that both large and small airways are narrowed. The size of airways obstruction appears to depend on the aetiology of a particular attack although there are suggestions that the smaller airways are more commonly involved in children than adults. Tests which measure expiratory flow will show a reduction which reverts completely to normal once the attack has ceased. Very sensitive tests such as closing volume or frequency dependence of compliance may detect significant abnormalities even in the asymptomatic child.

During an attack of asthma, distribution of inspired air can become uneven resulting in poor ventilation perfusion of the inspired gas in some areas of the lungs. If large areas become affected arterial hypoxaemia will occur. Administration of bronchial dilators by inhalation may reach only the already adequately ventilated zones thus causing only a marginal increase in ventilation, of little therapeutic effect.

The arterial PCO_2 during an attack of asthma in children is usually normal or decreased because of hyperventilation. An increased arterial PCO_2 indicates impending ventilatory failure and a need for urgent intensive treatment. During an attack, in addition to bronchoconstriction, intraluminal factors such as mucus secretion and oedema also operate and lead to complete obstruction of smaller airways. Thus the child breathing at high lung volume has to work hard to inspire because his respiratory muscles are at a mechanical disadvantage. He finds it difficult to inspire rather than to expire. As he deteriorates his cardiac output and oxygen consumption rise and due to the negative pressure within the chest there is an increase of the transluminal pressure on the left atrium and the pulmonary circulation. This course of events leads to a fall of the minute ventilation and results in distressed breathing pattern.

Despite the frequency of asthma, opportunities of examining pathological lung specimens are relatively uncommon. Most studies describe changes following an acute attack of asthma. The lungs are noted to be distended and small bronchi up to 1 mm in diameter are obstructed with thick plugs of mucus. The mucus is rich in glycoprotein and often Curschmann's spirals and Charcot–Leyden crystals of glycoproteins are seen. It is thought that the mucus originates from the submucus glands and the goblet cells. Many eosinophils and epithelial cells are also present. Microscopy of the bronchial wall shows an increase in the number of goblet cells and mucus glands and some shedding of the superficial epithelium. The basement membrane appears thick and contains eosinophils and lymphocytes. Very small bronchi often show squamous metaplasia as well as the thickening of the basement membrane. Such thickening may be demonstrated on biopsy specimens obtained during asymptomatic periods. The bronchial muscle is hypertrophied and at times areas of infection in the alveoli or in the surrounding tissues are present.

It is likely that with the development of fibreoptic bronchoscopy it will be possible to perform more frequent and detailed observations in some selected individuals with asthma.

Allergy

This is an important cause of attacks of asthma in the majority of children. Type I and Type III hypersensitivity reactions are involved but there is little evidence to support the involvement of Type II and IV reactions. Many other factors may be responsible for episodes of asthma and these include emotional disturbances, laughter, hyperventilation, viral or bacterial infections, weather conditions and non-specific irritants, e.g. smoke, chemicals and exercise. An increase in knowledge of these trigger factors has paved the way for better understanding of the disorder in children. However, the exact way such factors operate in producing bronchospasm is still uncertain.

Allergy and asthma: possible mechanisms

A number of theories have been put forward to explain how allergy may be involved in causing attacks of asthma. During the late 1960's it was suggested that asthmatic individuals had an excess of sympathetic constrictor alpha receptors on the smooth muscles of the airways and a relative reduction of the dilator beta receptors. This results in contraction of the smooth muscle following stimuli which in a healthy person are of little effect. Exciting though such a supposition may be, absolute proof is lacking.[3] Another speculative view states that inhaled allergens diffuse into the tissues of the respiratory tract where they act on mast cells causing the release of pharmacological mediators responsible for the bronchoconstriction.[5] There is a number of unanswered questions concerned with this theory such as the different sizes of allergens and lack of proof that any allergens are absorbed by the bronchial capillaries.

The most recent hypothesis states that allergens combine with antibodies on the surface of the bronchial epithelial cells and cause the release of chemical mediators which in turn act on the nervous receptors in these cells, thus evoking a reflex bronchoconstriction by way of the afferent and efferent pathways in the vagus nerve.[5-7,9] Supportive evidence for this observation both in animals and man is available. For instance, albumin sensitised dogs develop bronchoconstriction as part of an anaphylactic reaction. The bronchoconstriction can be abolished by a vagotomy or an injection of atropine. In man atropine by injection or in aerosol form can prevent attacks of asthma and inhibit allergen induced bronchoconstriction. Local anaesthetic vagal blockade is equally effective.[8] It would appear that vagal parasympathetic reflex mechanisms may very well be responsible for some degree of bronchoconstriction in some subjects with asthma.

Type I allergy

This reaction is mediated by the IgE antibody and occasionally by the IgG sensitising antibody. Initially the child becomes sensitised by the inhalation and absorption of small amounts of allergens over a period of time. These allergens then stimulate the production of IgE and IgG antibodies. IgE antibodies are produced by plasma cells and are known to sensitise blood tissue basophils and mast cells throughout the body. Such sensitised cells are capable of reacting with specific allergens because of the IgE antibodies which are fixed to mast cells and causes their degranulation and the release of chemical mediators such as the histamine, slow reacting substance of anaphylaxis, bradykinin, prostaglandins and the eosinophilic chaemotactic factor.[1]

It should be pointed out that there is little experimental evidence that in man inhalation of allergens does consistently cause degranulation of mast cells and the release of specific mediators. However, it is known that mast cells are present in the bronchial epithelium and may become degranulated during an acute attack of asthma provoked by non-specific factors.[10] It is also likely that the globule leucocytes which are present in the bronchial epithelium and contain granules may be involved in immunological reactions.[11]

The concentrations of IgE in the serum of healthy children ranges from 0·1–0·7 i.u./ml (plasma ± 125 i.u./ml). It has a molecular weight of 200,000 and sediments at 8·2. In common with IgG, papain digestion breaks the molecule into two (Fab) fragments carrying the antibody combining sites and crystalline piece (Fc). Both ends of the IgE antibody make an important contribution to its functional properties. It is the Fc end of the immunoglobulin that binds to the mast cells and basophils and about 10,000–40,000 molecules become attached to each cell. As the antibody combining sites are not involved in cellular attachment they are free to combine with antigen and if two or more molecules are crosslinked by allergen, histamine is released from the cells. Histamine is also released if the cross-linking is effected by an anti-IgE.

Serum IgE levels are raised in atopic diseases in childhood. A nonallergic child will show insignificant rises of serum IgE. In one study of 197 children 47 per cent were observed to have raised concentrations. Those children sensitive to two or more allergens had a higher incidence of raised levels of IgE serum (52 per cent) than those reacting to one allergen (23 per cent). Higher levels of IgE are obtained with food allergy and in children with atopic dermatitis and urticaria. A course of hyposensitisation has a minimal stimulatory effect on serum IgE concentrations as well as IgG and IgA.[12] During pollen seasons, high levels of IgE are obtained which revert to normal values during the winter months. This finding demonstrates that IgE has a very short half-life and that it becomes synthesised in the presence of an antigen. In general the degree of increase of serum IgE bears little clinical relevance to the intensity of the hypersensitivity state so that a child may have a normal serum IgE level yet be capable of mounting a considerable hypersensitivity reaction.

Type III allergy

IgG precipitating antibodies may be responsible for producing Type III allergic asthma but they should be distinguished from the IgE anaphylactic antibodies. These produce damage by means of the release of pharmacological substances like histamine, while IgG precipitins produce damage mediated by antigen–antibody complexes and complement. It is worth stressing that Type III allergic asthma is uncommon in children.

Late skin and bronchial challenge reactions

The late skin reaction consists of erythema and induration which develops at the site of the immediate hypersensitivity reaction about 3 to 5 hours after the initial response has disappeared.[13] The skin reactions are dose related, i.e. the larger the antigen used for immediate reaction the more likely is a later reaction observed. Although some attribute these late reactions to Type III hypersensitivity it is likely that they are IgE mediated because they appear to be dose related and systemic features such as leucocytosis or pulmonary infiltrates are absent.[14,15] The commonest allergens to which late skin reactions are obtained are the *Dermatophagoides pteronyssinus,* house dust, grass and ragweed pollens, animal epithelia, moulds, *Aspergillus fumigatus* and feathers.

Late bronchial reactions consist of bronchoconstriction commencing after an interval of a few hours following antigen challenge, i.e. usually 4 to 6 hours. The reactions may last for 24 to 48 hours. As with skin reactions, although features are compatible with Type III allergy, definite proof is lacking. Nevertheless, some children develop feverish episodes and leucocytosis which may possibly be attributed to impurities of the allergens. Dual bronchial reactions are characteristic following the inhalation of extract of *Aspergillus fumigatus* and are most common following the inhalation of the house dust mite, house dust and animal epithelia. These findings are clinically relevant especially in those children who predominantly develop nocturnal symptoms. In general, a positive late skin reaction to an allergen also implies bronchial hypersensitivity to that allergen.[16,17] Also clinically important is the demonstration that both the immediate and late reactions can be effectively blocked by prior administration of sodium cromoglycate while corticosteroids (oral or aerosol) block the late reactions only (Fig. 8.1).

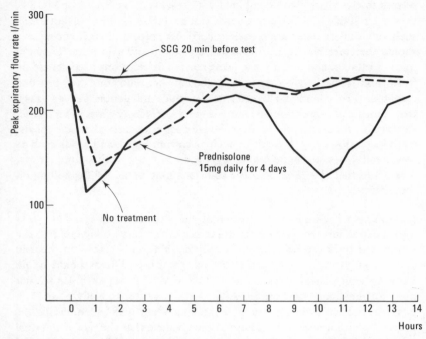

Fig. 8.1 Bronchial challenge tests to *D. pteronyssinus* in a boy, demonstrating immediate and late reactions, full protection by SCG, prevention of the late reaction only by prednisolone

Diagnosis

Diagnosis of IgE mediated asthma is based on history and physical examination, demonstration of IgE antibodies and blood eosinophilia. The most important aspect is positive history which will not only establish the diagnosis but also give a clue to the possible allergens which may be of aetiological significance. Physical examination may show chest deformities or occasionally minor bronchospasm and evidence of other atopic states such as eczema or rhinitis. Blood eosinophilia, although not always present, is a valuable finding and usually ranges from 400–800 eosinophils/mm³ (5–10 per cent of the total differential count).

Skin tests

These form a useful aid to the diagnosis. Skin tests measure the response of the skin to challenge by various antigens, but they may not necessarily be related to the response of bronchial mucosa nor need they be related to the mechanism producing the actual illness. If carried out correctly related to the history and combined with tests such as RAST or PRIST, they are reliable. The skin responses can be suppressed by certain drugs such as antihistamines and possibly corticosteroids and such substances should therefore be withheld for 48 hours before any skin tests. The only tests of value in children are the prick tests. The solutions used should be fresh and contain allergens in sufficient concentration to provoke response. The common allergens used include inhalants such as grass, tree, shrub and flower pollens, moulds such as *cladosporium, penicillium, Aspergillus fumigatus,* house dust, house dust mite, animal dander, birds' feathers, various vegetable fibres such as cotton, kapok and foods such as cow's milk, casein, lactalbumin, egg yolk and egg white, nuts, fruits, meats and fish. To this list other solutions may be added depending on the history.

Method. No preliminary cleansing of the skin is required. The volar aspect of the forearm is the best site to use but in very young children the skin of the back can be utilised. A drop of solution is placed on the skin and the skin pricked by needle through the drop. There should be no bleeding which invalidates the test. The method is very similar to that used for smallpox vaccination. After a few minutes, usually 5 to 15, a positive reaction is demonstrated by an area of erythema surrounding the prick site with a weal in the centre. Some believe that the size of the weal relates to the degree of hypersensitivity. The weal and flare reaction disappears after 30 minutes to 2 hours except in those children who show late responses. The size of reactions should be measured in mm only. A coding of reactions as + or ++ is subjective, inaccurate and of little value.

Bronchial provocation tests

Solutions for the test are the same as for skin tests although it is possible to omit the phenol preservative which may irritate bronchial mucosa. No drugs of any sort should be administered for at least 24 hours before a test which should be carried out during a full remission. Pulmonary function tests should be performed such as FEV_1, FVC and peak expiratory flow rates (PEFR). A nebuliser is used starting with a small dose of an allergen and increasing the concentration gradually, making sure to avoid any non-specific irritation of the respiratory epithelium. Positive results are shown by bronchial constriction and hypersecretion, cough and reduction of 20 per cent or more of FEV_1, FVC or PEFR. Occasionally allergic rhinitis may develop during a test and after a period of a few hours, pulmonary and nasal eosinophilia. Only one allergen is used at any one time and on any one day. Often bronchial challenge tests require termination with bronchodilators because of the severity of response.

Nasal provocation tests are occasionally used by employing one nostril for a test and using the other one as control. A drop of test solution is placed in one nostril. Positive reactions usually arise within a few minutes and there is mucosal reddening, swelling, hypersecretion and occasionally sneezing. One test is performed daily. On occasions an attack of asthma may be provoked.

Specific precipitating antibodies

These antibodies may be found in the sera of some children who are sensitive to birds such as pigeons, budgerigars, parrots, and to *Aspergillus fumigatus* and other moulds. Although Type I reactions in the skin may be observed at times, often they are not. The presence of these antibodies supports Type III hypersensitivity, most likely mediated by IgG antibodies.

The radioallergosorbent test (RAST)

This test is allergen and IgE specific. The test, similar in principle to the indirect Coombs' test for the detection of antibodies to red blood cells in the sera of Rh negative women, is based on the fact that allergens of different types can be chemically coupled to a CNBr-activated polymer either Sephadex or cellulose particles or filter paper discs which retain their capacity to bind antibodies of the IgE class. When such antibodies are bound they can further bind anti-IgE antibodies which can be purified and labelled with radioactive isotopes. The quantity of radioactivity is related to the amount of IgE in the serum (Fig. 8.2). The test is straightforward, rapid but expensive. A hundred or more tests can be performed daily.

So far RAST has been used to estimate IgE antibodies in sera to foods such as cow's milk, egg white, fish and nuts, pollens, house dust and house dust mites, animal epithelia, moulds, stinging insects and penicillin.

The test correlates well with the results of bronchial provocation tests (90–96 per cent) moderately well with skin tests (60–85 per cent) and leucocyte histamine release tests. RAST correlates poorly with blood eosinophilia. Sera can be stored almost indefinitely at 20°C until analysed and results obtained within 24 hours.[1,18–21]

Lung function tests

These are best related to the child's body size rather than age because

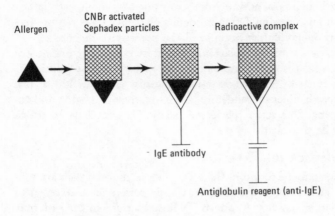

Fig. 8.2 The principle of radioallergosorbent test (RAST) for the measurement of specific IgE antibody

children of similar age vary in size. Tests performed randomly are of no clinical value and may be misleading. The majority of the available tests can have wide variations in normal values, on average ± 15 per cent about the mean. It is important, therefore, to calibrate the equipment periodically, determine one's own normal values especially for BTPS (body, temperature, pressure with 100 per cent water saturation) and employ a number of tests to assess lung function.

A child of 6 years and older can be fully studied. Most difficulties arise with younger children although many 3-, 4- and 5-year-olds co-operate in using a Wright's peak flow meter (low range model). More specialised tests such as the measurement of the functional residual capacity and body plethysmography to assess airway resistance are only occasionally indicated in asthmatic children. For details of the methods and interpretation of results the reader is referred elsewhere.[24,25]

Exercise as diagnostic test

A useful physiological classification of asthma based on exercise testing has been developed.[28] The FEV_1 or peak expiratory flow rate (PEFR) is measured at rest. These parameters are remeasured following an exercise of 6 to 8 minutes duration. Observations are continued until values return to normal. At this stage isoprenaline aerosol is administered for 3 minutes in 9 l of oxygen followed by a brisk 2 minute exercise. Measurements are made until values return to normal (usually within 20 minutes). The differences between the high and low values for FEV_1 are then expressed as percentage of the predicted normal.

$$\text{Lability index} = \frac{\text{Fall of } FEV_1 + \text{Rise of } FEV_1}{\text{Predicted normal } FEV_1} \times 100$$

With rare exceptions an asthmatic child has a Lability Index (L.I.) of well over 20 per cent. The majority (over 80 per cent) have a L.I. of between 20 and 30 per cent. Between 5 and 20 per cent of children have low FEV_1 values at rest, i.e. below the predicted normal for age and variable L.I. But usually between 30 and 50 per cent. With age the L.I. has a tendency towards normality but in the majority of asthmatic children it still remains abnormal although clinical attacks of asthma have ceased. The test therefore, is diagnostic and of prognostic value although long-term studies are so far lacking (Table 8.1).

Table 8.1 The fate of Lability Index in 67 asthmatic children*

	Initial	Final
Group 1	39	35
Group 2	28	27
Normal	—	5

* Assessed between 14 and 17 years, symptom free for 5 years (39 boys, 28 girls).

Running on a flat surface or a treadmill or brisk walking are the best type of exercises whereas swimming and cycling give unreliable results. A normal child (or very occasionally an asthmatic child) may show a post-exercise fall in FEV_1 or PEFR of about 5–10 per cent;[26] if it is more than that asthma should be suspected and if more than 15–20 per cent the diagnosis is almost certain. The exercise test is a simple everyday procedure and bronchodilators to terminate occasional bronchoconstriction are rarely required.

Recently a number of cheap and reliable devices have been produced such as the peak-flow gauge or the Airflometer which correlates well with the peak expiratory flow rate and FEV_1. The instruments give reproducible results although there may be as much as ± 10 per cent standard deviation between individual devices and unreliable measurements obtained at low flow rates. Thus assessments should always be made with the same instrument which can be used to study the L.I. and the response to any treatment.[27]

Undoubtedly the daily recording of symptoms and once or twice daily simple objective measurements of lung function are the ideals in management and should form a part of routine care of the asthmatic child (Fig. 8.3). There is evidence that at times the severity of asthma may be underestimated by the patient, parent or the doctor and one way of preventing serious delay in seeking urgent treatment is to utilize such objective measurements of lung function at home.

Instructions: Every evening ring round the nearest description of how your child has been and write in how many Intal Spincaps he has taken. You can, if you wish, add up the total scores of each day as an easy guide to his progress.

	Day	1	2	3	4	5	6	7	8	9	10
Number of Spincaps taken that day—											
COUGH	None	0	0	0	0	0	0	0	0	0	0
	Occasional	1	1	1	1	1	1	1	1	1	1
	Often	2	2	2	2	2	2	2	2	2	2
WHEEZE	None	0	0	0	0	0	0	0	0	0	0
	Occasional	1	1	1	1	1	1	1	1	1	1
	Often	2	2	2	2	2	2	2	2	2	2
ENERGY	Usual self	0	0	0	0	0	0	0	0	0	0
	Easily tired	1	1	1	1	1	1	1	1	1	1
	Mostly inactive	2	2	2	2	2	2	2	2	2	2
PLAY/GAMES	Normal	0	0	0	0	0	0	0	0	0	0
	Slight cough and/or wheeze	1	1	1	1	1	1	1	1	1	1
	Severe cough and/or wheeze	2	2	2	2	2	2	2	2	2	2
MEALS	Usual self	0	0	0	0	0	0	0	0	0	0
	Some interest	1	1	1	1	1	1	1	1	1	1
	No interest	2	2	2	2	2	2	2	2	2	2
SLEEP	Normal	0	0	0	0	0	0	0	0	0	0
	Mildly disturbed	1	1	1	1	1	1	1	1	1	1
	Poor night	2	2	2	2	2	2	2	2	2	2
	TOTAL SCORE										

REMARKS

Fig. 8.3 Daily record card. (Reproduced by permission of Fisons Ltd.)

Differential diagnosis

It is important to exclude by appropriate investigations cystic fibrosis, hypogammaglobulinaemia, alpha₁ antitrypsin deficiency, bronchiectasis, chronic adenoidal infection, foreign bodies in bronchus, congenital heart disease and external compressions of the trachea by enlarged lymph nodes or vascular anomalies.

Complications of asthma in children

Status asthmaticus is the most common and the most serious;

Pulmonary collapse-consolidation;

Chest deformities, e.g. pigeon chest, barrel-chest, Harrison's sulcus;

Pulmonary eosinophilic infiltrations, e.g. *Aspergillus fumigatus*;[22,23]

Bronchiectasis;

Pneumothorax;

Spontaneous emphysema;

Cor pulmonale;

Compensatory polycythaemia.

Management

Treatment of the asthmatic child can be usefully considered under two headings:

a. To provide relief of symptoms;
b. To minimise or prevent the future development of attacks.

Management of an acute attack

Some minor attacks will cease spontaneously following a period of rest. Adrenaline still remains the most effective drug. An s.c. injection of a solution of adrenaline 1:1000 should be given slowly in a dose of 0·01 mg/kg body weight up to a volume of 0·3 ml. The child's progress should be observed for 30 minutes. The majority of children will improve significantly during that time and additional treatment can be continued with an oral bronchodilator. If the child fails to improve and provided he has not developed tachycardia of more than 160/min, a second dose of adrenaline can be given. Failure to respond to the second dose of adrenaline is a clear indication of admission to hospital. In certain situations terbutaline as an s.c. injection of 0·1 mg/kg up to the maximum dose of 0·25 mg/kg may be useful. Its duration of action is about 4 hours.

In a very small child some attacks can be terminated by the use of aminophylline suppository (5 mg/kg) and subsequent treatment continued with an oral bronchodilator. Aminophylline can be given i.v. to the older child (4 mg/kg) and if so it should be given very slowly, i.e. over 10 to 15 minutes. Oral bronchodilators, xanthine derivatives and other sympathomimetics should be discontinued as soon as bronchoconstriction has been completely reversed and certainly not employed for longer than

2 to 4 days. Indiscriminate and prophylactic use of the various symptomatic agents makes little therapeutic sense and should be condemned. It is worth pointing out that some bronchodilator drugs exert profound effects on mucus synthesis and glycoprotein secretion, e.g.—adrenergic agents have variable actions; methylxanthines cause significant increases. Since our knowledge of the physiology and biochemistry of bronchial secretions is little known, prolonged therapeutic stimulus of these secretions may, in the long run, be of disadvantage to the patient.[38-40]

Oral corticosteroids for acute attacks at home

If the child has not responded relatively quickly to a parenteral bronchodilator he should either be admitted to hospital for further management or he should be given corticosteroids immediately and his progress assessed every few hours. Before corticosteroids are administered at home it is essential to make sure that the family can cope, and understand all the instructions which should be clearly written down. They should be instructed to call the doctor back immediately should the child deteriorate, or failing to locate him, to take the child to the nearest hospital.

General measures

It is important to maintain good hydration by insisting on sufficient oral intake of fluids. The asthmatic child may become dehydrated because of increased work of breathing and insensible fluid loss through the lungs, or he may have had diuresis if xanthines have been used. Adequate hydration prevents accumulation of thick secretions and thus may partly prevent pulmonary collapse. It is important to write down exact instructions for the parents and review the child's progress in 4 to 6 hours. If the oral intake of fluids should for any reason be inadequate, the child should be admitted to hospital as i.v. therapy will be required.

The use of antihistamines and mucolytic agents is contra-indicated in acute attacks of asthma because they have a tendency to dry up the secretions and enhance plugging of thick mucus. Sedatives are also contra-indicated because they can cause respiratory depression and mask hypoxaemia. If there is a large element of anxiety then chloral hydrate is the safest to use. If there is a possibility of infection an antibiotic should be given.

Treatment of status asthmaticus

A child should be considered to be in status asthmaticus if his acute attack has failed to show sustained improvement within 2 or 3 hours or has failed to respond to adequate doses of parenteral bronchodilators.

A full assessment of the child should be done immediately on admission. Oxygen therapy with humidity should be started at once and blood obtained for electrolytes, urea, haematological values and gas analysis. An i.v. drip should be set up and a portable X-ray obtained to exclude pneumothorax.

Many children will have metabolic acidosis which should be corrected by the administration of sodium bicarbonate slowly over a period of 15 to 30 minutes. The administration of sodium bicarbonate can be calculated according to the Astrup formula (base deficit $\times 0.3 \times$ body weight in kg = m-mol required for complete correction). The value of sodium bicarbonate is to enhance the action of adrenaline on bronchial smooth muscle which is known to be reduced in states of acidosis. It is unnecessary to correct pH above 7.3.

If the child has not had aminophylline during the previous 24 hours and is adequately hydrated, i.v. aminophylline should be given (5 mg/kg) as a constant infusion during a 4 to 6 hour period. It is essential to estimate theophylline blood levels regularly as a guide to efficient treatment and in order to avoid any possible toxic effects. The therapeutic level of theophylline is between 10–20 μg/ml and serious side-effects are uncommon if theophylline level is below 20 μg/ml.[29]

About 30 to 60 minutes should be allowed to assess the response to initial treatment which will have included oxygen, aminophylline, fluids and i.v. sodium bicarbonate. If the child has shown a definite clinical improvement a trial of nebulised salbutamol may be started provided his pulse rate is less than 160/min. The use of nebulised salbutamol may be helpful in some situations although some young children become frightened by the mask as they feel a sense of choking. Nebulised therapy is of much practical value for terminating minor episodes of asthma provided a suitable compressor is available, i.e. to produce a flow rate of 4–5 l/min.

Corticosteroids. These should always be considered and there should be no hesitation in using corticosteroids if the child has had any steroid treatment within the previous 3 months or so. Corticosteroids should be used very early following admission rather than later as it takes a number of hours for their full effect to become apparent. When in doubt it is safer to use them rather than wait. The appropriate dose is hydrocortisone (5 mg/kg) given i.v. every 4 hours as a continuous infusion after an initial loading dose of 5 mg/kg. If the child is able to take corticosteroids orally, prednisolone 2 mg/kg should be given every 4 hours until clinical improvement occurs, after which time they can be discontinued very rapidly.

If the child is restless, has tachycardia and a rising $PaCo_2$ and low

PaO$_2$ progress should be discussed with an anaesthetist as assisted ventilation may be necessary. Bronchial lavage is rarely required in asthmatic children. Assisted mechanical ventilation is not without risks. (Subcutaneous emphysema, pneumothorax and laryngeal stenosis due to intubation.) It should not be considered lightly in any child. The best guide for considering assisted ventilation is progressive fatigue of the child and a gradual rise of PaCo$_2$ to about 55–65 mmHg. Single or infrequent values of PaCo$_2$ should be interpreted with great caution.

Physiotherapy. This should be started when a definite clinical improvement has occurred. Frequent postural drainage is helpful as it facilitates the removal of secretions and opening of small airways.

Long-term management

Following recovery from an acute attack of asthma full assessment should be carried out and should include details of the family and past history, haematology, L.I., skin tests, RAST etc.

Whatever subsequent treatment is decided upon it is useful to keep a daily record card of symptoms and a twice daily record of the expiratory flow rates for the next 4 weeks. It is of immense value to keep a record for 2 or 3 weeks before any active treatment is used. Such observations serve as a base line and give subjective and objective data which can be used for comparing responses to any therapy.

Bronchodilators

If the attacks are infrequent, mild in nature and do not interfere with the child's activities, periodic administration of a bronchodilator such as salbutamol or terbutaline is all that is required. It is useful to write clear instructions for the parents. Many children are prescribed bronchodilators unnecessarily and prophylactically for indefinite periods between infrequent attacks. At times two or three bronchodilators are used simultaneously, such polypharmacy is to be condemned. It is far better to use one established bronchodilator which the doctor knows best rather than to use fashionable agents of doubtful additional therapeutic value.

Methylxanthines are also useful for such minor episodes provided laboratory facilities for blood analyses are available because significant variations in dose responses and drug elimination occur between children. Thus it is important to determine an adequate therapeutic dose for each child (4–10 mg/kg per 24 hr). Satisfactory blood theophylline levels lie between 10 and 20 μg/ml. Prophylactic use of theophylline should only be considered if laboratory facilities for drug estimation are available as often much larger doses are needed to control symptoms, e.g. 20–30 mg/kg per 24 hr.[30] Theophylline has a half life of 2 to 4 hours in children over 3 to 6 months of age, hence needs to be given often to be therapeutically effective. The use of combinations of methylxanthines and bronchodilators should be discouraged as such combinations may lead to the early appearance of side-effects.

Sodium cromoglycate

Recurrent episodes of asthma associated with allergy are best prevented by sodium cromoglycate. It acts by stablising mast cell membranes thus inhibiting the release of the various pharmacological mediators responsible for bronchospasm. Numerous studies during the last 10 years have confirmed the beneficial effects of this agent in children. About 80 per cent of children respond effectively to sodium cromoglycate. It is a prophylactic agent and should be administered regularly, every day and over a long period of time. Apart from occasional dryness of the throat and cough after inhalation it appears to be free from serious side-effects. Each capsule contains 20 mg of sodium cromoglycate in a lactose base. Following inhalation about 10 per cent of the drug is retained in the spinhaler, 30–50 per cent deposited in the mouth, 10 per cent enters the bronchi and lungs and the rest is swallowed and appears unchanged in faeces. Only about 4 per cent of the drug is actually absorbed in the lungs.

The majority of children over the age of 3 years can inhale sodium cromoglycate effectively provided the doctor takes time and patience to teach the child and his mother how to use the spin-haler correctly. The dosage of sodium cromoglycate is one capsule 4 times daily for the first month or longer. Once the child's progress becomes satisfactory the dose can be reduced to 3 or 2 capsules a day. On occasions children who do not respond to 2 or 4 capsules a day will improve when the dose is increased to 6 capsules daily.

Some infants, too young to use spin-halers can benefit by using sodium cromoglycate in a nebulised form. However helpful such an approach, it is much more successful in a hospital setting than at home because it is often difficult to obtain the child's undivided attention during each treatment for many minutes.

Steroid aerosols

If the child is not obtaining significant benefit from sodium cromoglycate or bronchodilators, it is rational to try the effect of steroid aerosols such as beclomethasone diproprionate or betametasone 17 valerate. The mode of action of glucocorticosteroids in asthma is not fully understood. They may act by reducing the inflammatory responses and thus inhibiting the mediators of inflammation or by sensitising the beta adrenergic receptors to catecholamine stimulation and promoting the formation of cyclic AMP.

Following each inhalation only about 10 per cent of the drug actually reaches the lungs. The aerosols are dispensed in pressurised canisters containing approximately 200 doses and each puff delivers 50 or 100 μg respectively. The dose in children is two puffs (100 and 200 μg) respectively 2 to 4 times a day. Many studies have demonstrated the beneficial effects of steroid aerosols in children with chronic asthma, the steroid dependent and those poorly controlled with other agents.

The only significant side-effect is the occasional transient hoarseness and localised colonisation of the nasopharynx with *Candida albicans*, growth of which is dose related, i.e. the incidence is higher when 800 μg per day of steroid aerosol are given than when the dose is 400 μg or less.

Corticosteroids and corticotrophin

There is a number of children who do not derive sufficient relief of symptoms from either sodium cromoglycate or steroid aerosols but respond to oral corticosteroids. If possible such children should receive intermittent therapy (e.g. prednisolone 2 mg/kg) in order to minimise the suppression of the hypothalamo–pituitary–adrenal axis, thus reducing the incidence of the numerous side-effects especially the stunting of growth. In all such children, it is important to assess periodically the state of the hypothalamo–pituitary–adrenal system by the tetracosactrin screening tests.[1]

ACTH is an alternative to oral corticosteroids. It is of most value as a short-term measure because of the disadvantage of having to be injected. The dose may vary between 10 and 80 units daily.

All children on corticosteroids should always carry a steroid warning card.

Newer anti-asthma agents

A number of orally effective agents similar in action to sodium cromoglycate is being developed for the prophylactic treatment of asthma (see page 79). One of these, ketotifen[41] possesses anti-anaphylactic and antihistaminic properties. Preliminary clinical studies are few, indefinite but encouraging. None of the newer agents however, has so far been shown to be superior to sodium cromoglycate or steroid aerosols.

Immunotherapy

The indications and rationale have been fully discussed on pages 74–79.

If the history and investigations strongly suggest that exposure to allergens is causing exacerbations of the child's asthma one should fully discuss with parents the best possible means of avoiding or reducing contact with the allergens concerned (see page 71). One of the simplest preventive measures is to ensure adequate humidification of the bedroom air if the house is fully centrally heated.

Before immunotherapy is recommended one should consider the age of the child, his previous response to drug treatment and the real possibility that he may not derive benefit from a prolonged course of injections which may also cause anaphylactic reactions. The best results from hyposensitisation are obtained in those children who suffer from seasonal asthma. There are only a few long prospective studies of the value of hyposensitisation in children. In one study with a follow-up of 14 years the best results were obtained in children with perennial asthma (71 per cent) who had received high concentrations of allergens.[36]

When hyposensitisation is used for seasonal asthma it is essential to time the course of injections so that the last one is given shortly before the season commences. A number of carefully conducted studies have shown that if hyposensitisation is properly carried out, the majority of subjects will show significant improvement (Table 8.2). For details of doses and course of treatment please see pages 76–78.

House dust and asthma

Although the majority of children will give positive reactions to the house dust mite on skin testing with RAST and bronchial provocation tests, we have not been convinced that a short course of hyposensitisation is of significant benefit in asthmatic children. Although hyposensitisation may lower or even abolish hypersensitive reaction to the house dust mite in the skin, it does not appear to coincide with the improvement of the child's asthma. There are indications that if the injections are continued for a long time, perhaps years, better results can be obtained.

Psychological status

The study of the psychological background of the asthmatic child is beneficial in long-term management. There is little doubt that many minor episodes are precipitated by psychosomatic factors. One is also impressed by the fact that with proper attitude and management of these minor attacks, the psychological state of both the child and his family considerably improves. Nevertheless, on occasions psychiatric problems do occur and require a child psychiatrist's help.

Some children who lack confidence in themselves, and are anxious and insecure may benefit from hypnotherapy. After all, suggestion plays an

Table 8.2 Hyposensitisation and asthma

Reference	Year	Allergens	Active treatment	Placebo	% improvement	
					Treated	Placebo
31	1954	Grass pollens	100	89	78	34
32	1971	House dust mite	11	11	91	27
33	1971	House dust	52	28	87	32
34	1973	House dust Grass pollens etc.	10	5	80	15
35	1973	House dust mite	45	46	75	64
38	1974	House dust mite	41	21	38	4

important part in many forms of medical treatment and its efficacy can be exploited for the relief of asthmatic symptoms. Hypnosis should be considered as an adjunct to other forms of treatment and should be practiced by the doctor who treats the child's asthma. A doctor who has no working experience of hypnosis is missing an opportunity of being able to help some of his young patients. For details of patient selection, methods of induction and the phenomena of hypnosis, the reader is referred elsewhere.[37]

Breathing exercises and physical fitness exercises

Breathing exercises may help the asthmatic child to relax and if he and his parents are convinced of their benefit then they should be encouraged, but never insisted upon. Undoubtedly breathing exercises improve ventilation and correct postural deformities. Some children also derive psychological advantages from such exercises thus relieving anxiety and gaining confidence.

Many asthmatic children do not participate in games especially at school for fear of precipitating an attack. It is important to discuss this aspect with the mother, the child and the teacher. In the majority of cases bronchoconstriction can be almost completely prevented by the prior administration of a bronchodilator such as salbutamol which should be taken 20 minutes before exercise or games. Other drugs may be equally successful. Steroid aerosols and corticosteroids have no demonstrable effects on exercise induced bronchoconstriction. Short exercises such as swimming and short games are tolerated well. Singing lessons are of immense value.

Asthma and immunisations

Smallpox vaccination is contra-indicated in children with eczema, septic skin or recurrent rashes or who live with children suffering from similar disorders. Most of the immunisations are well tolerated. If the child is egg sensitive then a dog, chick or rabbit cell culture vaccine should be employed.

Asthma and operations

Anaesthetic procedures are well tolerated in the asthmatic child. However, if he has received corticosteroids during the previous 3 months, cortisone injection BP (2 mg/kg) should be given 6 hourly for 24 hours by i.m. injections for minor operations and 72 hours or longer for a major operation. In acute emergencies hydrocortisone hemisuccinate (2 mg/kg) should be given i.v. as a single injection and subsequently a course of cortisone injections should be employed.

References

1. Kuzemko, J. A. (1976) Asthma in Children. Tunbridge Wells: Pitman Medical.
2. Turner-Warick, M. (1977) On observing patterns of airflow obstruction in chronic asthma. *Br. J. dis. Chest*, **71**, 73.
3. Blair, H. (1977) Natural history of childhood asthma: 20 year follow up. *Archs dis. Child.*, **52**, 613.
4. Gold, W. M. (1975) The role of the parasympathetic nervous system in airways disease. *Postgrad. Med. J.*, **51** (Suppl. 7) 53.
5. Lichtenstein, L. M. (1973) *Asthma: Physiology, Immunopharmacology and Treatment*, p. 91. New York: Academic Press.
6. Empey, D. W., Laitinen, L. A., Jacobs, L., Gold, W. M. and Nadel, J. A. (1976) Mechanisms of bronchial hyperreactivity in normal subjects after upper respiratory tract infection. *Am. Rev. resp. Dis.*, **113**, 131.
7. Widdicombe, J. G. (1977) Some experimental models of acute asthma. *J. R. Coll. Phys.*, **II**, 2, 141.
8. Macklem, P. T. and Engel, L. A. (1975) The physiological complications of airways smooth muscle constriction. *Postgrad. Med. J.*, **51** (Suppl. 7) 45.
9. Widdicombe, J. G. (1975) Reflex control of airways of smooth muscle. *Postgrad. Med. J.*, **51** (Suppl. 7) 36.
10. Salvato, G. (1961) Mast cells in bronchial connective tissue in man. *Int. archs Allergy appl. Immunol.*, **18**, 348.
11. Jeffrey, P. K. and Reid, L. (1975) New observation of rat airway epithelium: a quantative and electronmicroscopic study. *J. Anatomy*, **120**, 295.
12. Deuschl, H., Johansson, S. G. O. and Fagerberg, E. (1977) IgE, IgG and IgA antibodies in serum and nasal secretion during parenteral hyposensitisation. *Clin. Allergy*, **7**, 315.
13. Praüsnitz, C. and Küstner, H. (1921) Studien über die Überempfindlichkeit. *CblH Bakteriol.*, **86**, 160.
14. Solley, G. O., Gleich, G. J., Jordan, R. E. and Schroeter, A. L. (1976) The late phase of the immediate weal and flare skin reaction. *J. clin. Invest.*, **58**, 408.
15. Zettersrom, O. (1978) Dual skin test reactions and serum antibodies to subtilisin and *Aspergillus fumigatus* extracts. *Clin. Allergy*, **8**, 77.
16. Warner, J. O. (1976) Significance of late reactions after bronchial challenge with house dust mite. *Archs dis. Child.*, **51**, 905.
17. Kerrebijn, F. J., Degenhart, H. J. and Hammers, A. (1976) Relation between skin tests, inhalation tests, and histamine release from leucocytes and IgE in house dust mite allergy. *Archs dis. Child.*, **51**, 252.
18. Gleich, G. J. and Yunginger, J. W. (1975) The radioallergosorbent test: Its present place and likely future in the practice of allergy. *Adv. Asthma Allergy*, **2**, 1.
19. Johansson, S. G. O. (1975) Determination of IgE and IgE antibody by RAST. In: *Advances in Diagnosis of Allergy: RAST*, p. 1. Miami: Richard Evans.
20. Johansson, S. G. O. (1975) Comparison of *in vivo* and *in vitro* tests for diagnosis of immediate hypersensitivity. In: *Laboratory Diagnosis of Immunological Disorders*. Ed. by Vyas, G. N., Stites, D. P. and Brechner, G., p. 225. New York: Stratton.
21. Aas, K. (1975) Diagnosis of immediate type respiratory allergy. *Pediatr. Clin. N. Am.*, **2**, 33.
22. Berger, I., Phillips, W., Shenker, I. (1972) Pulmonary aspergillosis in childhood. *Clin. Pediatrics*, **11**, 178.
23. Imbeau, S. A., Cohen, M. and Reed, C. E. (1977) Allergic bronchopulmonary aspergillosis in infants. *Am. J. Dis. Child.*, **131**, 1127.
24. Cotes, J. E. (1968) *Lung Function: Assessment and Application in Medicine*, 2nd ed. Oxford: Blackwell Scientific.
25. Polgar, G. and Promadhat, V. (1971) *Techniques and Standards for Pulmonary Function Tests in Children*. Philadelphia: Saunders.

26. Burr, M. L., Eldridge, B. A. and Borysiovicz, L. K. (1974) Peak expiratory flow rates before and after exercise in school children. *Archs dis. Child.*, **49,** 923.

27. Thompson, P., Friedman, M. and Walker, S. R. (1977) The airflometer—A new device for assessing changes in respiratory function. *The Practitioner,* **219,** 251.

28. Jones, R. S., Wharton, M. J. and Buston, M. H. (1963) The place of physical exercise and bronchodilator drugs in the assessment of the asthmatic child. *Archs dis. Child,* **38,** 539.

29. Weinberger, M. (1978) Theophylline for treatment of asthma. *J. Pediatr.,* **92,** 1.

30. Wyatt, R., Weinberger, M. and Hendeles, L. (1978) Oral theophylline dosage for the management of chronic asthma. *J. Pediatr.,* **92,** 125.

31. Frankland, A. W. and Augustin, R. (1954) Prophylaxis of summer hay-fever and asthma. *Lancet,* **I,** 1055.

32. Smith, A. P. (1971) Hyposensitisation with *D. pteronyssinus* antigen. *Br. med. J.,* **IV,** 204.

33. Aas, K. (1971) Hyposensitisation in house dust allergy and asthma. *Acta Paediatr. Scand.,* **60,** 264.

34. Tuchinda, M. and Chai, H. (1973) Effect of immunotherapy in chronic asthmatic children. *J. Allergy Clin. Immunol.,* **51,** 131.

35. D'Souza, M. F. D., Pepys, J., Wells, I. D., Tai, E., Plamer, F., Overell, B. G., McGrath, I. T. and Megson, M. (1973) Hyposensitisation with *Dermatophagoides pteronyssinus* in house dust allergy: A controlled study of clinical and immunological effects. *Clin. Allergy,* **3,** 177.

36. Johnston, D. E. and Dutton, A. (1968) Value of hyposensitisation for asthma in children—a 14 year study. *Pediatrics,* **42,** 793.

37. Hartland, J. (1973) *Medical and Dental Hypnosis and its Clinical Applications.* 2nd ed. London: Bailliere Tindall.

38. Sturgess, J. and Reid, L. (1972) Secretory activity of the human bronchial mucous glands *in vitro. Exp. molec. Pathol.,* **16,** 362.

39. Reid, L. (1974) Histopathological aspects of bronchial secretion. *Scand. J. resp. Dis.* (Suppl.) **90,** 9.

40. Reid, L. (1974) Rheology—relation to the composition of sputum. *Scand. J. resp. Dis.* (Suppl.) **90,** 27.

41. Prophylaxis of asthma—a new approach. (1978) Meeting at the Royal College of Physicians, London (in press).

CHAPTER 9

Eyes

ALLERGIC REACTIONS OF the eyes are less common in children than in adults. The eyelids may be involved in contact dermatitis, angioedema and urticaria. The conjunctiva may be affected in pollenosis, angioedema, urticaria and in food allergy. Indeed, conjunctivitis may at times be the only clinical sign of food hypersensitivity. The eyelids, like other skin surfaces are often involved in allergic reactions. Oedema of the eyelids is a common occurrence because of the loose subcutaneous tissues and the ease with which the swelling can protrude forwards.

Immunological aspects

It is well known that IgE mediated reactions occur in conjunctiva and indeed the conjunctival sac has been used in the past as a method of testing for allergy. Immunological studies of children's tears showed the presence of IgA (average 17 mg/100 ml), IgG (average 14 mg/100 ml), and practically no IgM and IgE (average value 250 ng/ml—comparable average serum level was 2000 ng/ml). Regrettably IgE levels were not studied in allergic diseases.[1]

Typically, vasodilatation and oedema occurs. There is some evidence of production of local antibody formation within the eye. Anaphylactic reactions especially involving the uvea have also been described. Acute inflammation follows with uveitis and iridocyclitis, and petechial haemorrhages can be observed in the iris. Type IV reactions (delayed sensitivity) have been well described and may involve the eyelids, conjunctiva, uveal tract and cornea.[2–6]

It is worth remembering that following recovery from the initial sensitisation to an allergen, subsequent eye symptoms may be caused by antigens which have entered the body by different routes, e.g. oral, intravenous, etc. It would appear therefore, that the eye possesses a high degree of hypersensitivity and is able to respond to new allergens much earlier than other organs.

Examination of the eye

A detailed history should be obtained and in particular questions should be asked about the onset of symptoms, pain and discomfort. It is important to enquire about previous episodes, and any possible history of allergy within the family.

The eyelids, lid margins and eyelashes should be inspected first, then the bulbar conjunctiva and the tarsal plates. The lower lids are easily everted allowing thorough inspection of the conjunctiva. Examination of the upper tarsal plate is conveniently achieved by asking the child to close his eye, grasping gently the lashes with the fingers of the left hand and simultaneously applying a minor counter-pressure externally over the upper margin of the lid with a plastic or glass rod. It is always essential to examine the everted upper lid as cobblestone appearance may be the only sign of vernal conjunctivitis.

In all instances, ulceration of the cornea should be excluded by staining it with fluorescein using Rose Bengal drops or Flue-i-strips. Patches of ulceration, staining pink with Rose Bengal drops or green with fluorescein will be seen. Difficulty may occasionally arise in differentiating conjunctivitis from iritis. In conjunctivitis, vision is always normal. There is discomfort rather than acute pain. The pupil and iris are normal and the cornea is clear. In acute iritis, the eye-sight is always affected and pain is severe. The iris itself is 'muddy' and the pupils are small, irregular and non-reacting. Glaucoma is rare in children but may occasionally mimic acute iritis in its onset. Testing for increased intraocular tension will easily confirm the diagnosis. In some countries (Africa, the Middle and Far East) inclusion conjunctivitis, which is bilateral in 30 per cent of subjects, should be considered by detecting TRIC agent, chlamydia trachamatis. Diagnosis is most important as some antibiotic eye ointments are very effective.[7-9]

When in doubt regarding the exact nature of an eye condition, an ophthalmologist's opinion should be urgently sought.

Eye allergy may manifest itself as contact dermatitis from cosmetics, etc., allergic conjunctivitis and vernal kerato-conjunctivitis.

Allergic conjunctivitis

Symptoms may be associated with allergic rhinitis which occurs during the pollen season or in children subject to perennial rhinitis. The child will complain of itchiness of the eyes which he frequently rubs causing an increase of the oedema.

On examination the conjunctivae are red and swollen, and there is a clear, watery discharge. If the discharge is examined it will contain increased numbers of eosinophils.

Treatment should consist, if possible, of allergen avoidance. Efficient treatment of allergic rhinitis and topical application of sympathomimetic drops, e.g. xylometazoline hydrochloride or an aqueous solution of 2 per cent sodium cromoglycate BP. It is important not to use this solution in children sensitive to benzalkonium chloride as it forms one of the components of the presentation.

Vernal kerato-conjunctivitis (from L. *vernalis*—spring)

Vernal kerato-conjunctivitis is a recurrent bilateral inflammatory disease of the conjunctivae which in its most severe forms occurs during the summer months. The upper tarsal conjunctiva often shows a papillary hypertrophy giving a characteristic 'cobblestone' appearance. Changes on the lower tarsal conjunctiva are less marked. The main histological changes comprise infiltration by plasma cells, lymphocytes, eosinophils and other inflammatory cells, some collagen hyperplasia and proliferative and degenerative changes of the epithelium. At times the aggregations of inflammatory cells can be seen as white or yellow dots (Trantas' spots). After one month or so, collagen fibres are laid down subepithelialy, hyalinisation occurs, the hyperplasia extends upwards in a papillary fashion and the spaces between papillae become filled with epithelium forming cysts full of mucin. In between attacks, mast cells are seen and often eosinophils, but few other inflammatory cells. The papillary changes persist during remission.

The natural history is towards spontaneous recovery after 5 to 10 years, although scarring of the conjunctiva may remain.[10,11] The condition is often associated with atopy and in 75–80 per cent of children, a history of eczema and/or asthma will be present.[12] In one study 13 out of 35 patients were allergic to foods and one to dust exposure.[13] Symptoms are often at their worst during May and June but some children may be worse at any time of the year.

The history will suggest allergic conjunctivitis, but in addition there may be photophobia. Examination of the eyes may reveal palpebral involvement only. The tarsal plate of the upper eyelid will have a 'cobblestone' appearance because of thickening and hyperplasia of the conjunctiva. If the junction of cornea and sclera is affected, corneal erosions may occur, leading to permanent scarring and loss of vision.

Management

General measures include avoiding allergens such as foods and dust and the efficient treatment of any associated atopic disease. Immunotherapy has so far not been tried in this condition. In one study,[13] four subjects with grass pollen asthma and vernal conjunctivitis undergoing hyposensitisation showed worsening of eye symptoms and reduction of excess of the sticky mucus so typical of this condition. Corneal ulceration may be helped by adding 10 per cent acetyl cysteine to other topical agents, and corneal plaques (granular material containing glycoprotein probably derived from mucus) can be removed by superficial keratectomy.[14] Topical antibiotics should only be used in the presence of an infection.

Frequent administration of corticosteroid eye drops is often effective in controlling acute symptoms.[7] However, in view of the recurrent nature of the condition, over-use of corticosteroids may lead to serious side effects. There is evidence for instance that a 6 weeks' course may cause an increase in intraocular pressure of greater than 19 mmHg.[15] Formation of cataracts and an increased susceptibility to bacterial and viral infections are other well recognised complications. A suitable preparation is Gutt Predsol 0·025 per cent three or four times daily. If ineffective, potency can be increased.

The frequent applications of 2 per cent sodium cromoglycate BP eye drops has been found of therapeutic value. In a 2 week double blind study of 22 patients, significant improvement occurred in 18 patients who showed reduction in itching, watering and photophobia. Examination of the eyes demonstrated a reduction in inflammatory processes, disappearance of Trantas' spots but no change in the 'cobblestone' appearance. A further 2 year study of 61 patients showed that 18 per cent could be controlled on sodium cromoglycate alone, and 72 per cent required additional short courses of topical steroid treatment. Four patients developed troublesome eye irritation necessitating the distribution of treatment. Overall, the need for prolonged courses of topical corticosteroids was considerably reduced.[16-18]

It is worth emphasing that any eye drops should be administered correctly if best results are to be obtained. The child should be in a supine position and the drops placed in the upper fornix. Absorption is increased if the eyelids are open for 15 to 30 seconds.

References

1. McClellan, B. H., Whitney, C. R., Newman, L. P. and Allansmith, M. R. (1973) Immunoglobulins in tears. *Am. J. Ophthalmol.*, **76,** 89.
2. Theodore, F. H. and Schlossman, A. (1958) Ocular Allergy. Baltimore: Williams and Wilkins.
3. Zimmerman, L. E. and Silverstein, A. M. (1959) Experimental ocular hypersensitivity. Histopathologic observations. *Am. J. Ophthalmol.*, **48,** 447.
4. Meyers, R. L. and Pettit, T. H. (1975) Pathogenesis of experimental allergic uveitis induced by retinal rod outer segments and pigment epithelium. *J. Immunol.*, **114,** 1269.
5. McMaster, P. R., Wong, V. G., Owens, J. D. and Kyriakos, M. (1975) Prevention of experimental allergic uveitis: treatment with methotrexate. *Archs Ophthalmol.*, **93,** 835.

6. Hammer, H. (1974) Cellular hypersensitivity to uveal pigment confirmed by leucocyte migration tests in sympathetic ophthalmitis and the Vogt–Koyanagi–Harada Syndrome. *Br. J. Ophthalmol.*, **58**, 773.

7. Jones, B. R. (1961) Vernal conjunctivitis. *Trans. Ophthalmol. Soc. U.K.*, **81**, 367.

8. Jones, B. R. (1974) Laboratory tests for chlamydial infection: Their role in epidemiological studies of trachoma and its control. *Br. J. Ophthalmol.*, **58**, 438.

9. Darougar, S., Viswalingam, M., Treharne, J. D., Kinnison, J. R. and Jones, B. R. (1977) Treatment of TRIC infection of the eye with Rifampicin or chloramphenicol. *Brit. J. Ophthalmol.*, **61**, 255.

10. Duke-Elder, S. (1965) *System of Ophthalmology.* Vol. 8, part 1, p. 475. London: Kimpton.

11. Morgan, G. (1971) The pathology of vernal conjunctivitis. *Trans. Ophthalmol. Soc. U.K.*, **91**, 467.

12. Allansmith, M. and Frick, O. L. (1963) Antibodies to grass in vernal conjunctivitis. *J. Allergy*, **34**, 535.

13. Frankland, A. W. and Easty, D. (1971) Vernal kerato-conjunctivitis: an atopic disease. *Trans. Ophthalmol. Soc. U.K.*, **91**, 479.

14. Rice, N. S. C., Easty, D., Garner, A., Jones, B. R. and Tripathi, R. (1971) Vernal kerato-conjunctivitis and its management. *Trans. Ophthalmol. Soc. U.K.*, **91**, 483.

15. Kass, M. A., Kolker, A. E. and Becker, B. (1972) Chronic topical corticosteroid use simulating congenital glaucoma. *J. Pediatr.*, **81**, 1175.

16. Easty, D., Rice, N. S. C. and Jones, B. R. (1971) Disodium cromoglycate (Intal) in the treatment of vernal kerato-conjunctivitis. *Trans. Ophthalmol. Soc. U.K.*, **91**, 491.

17. Easty, D., Rice, N. S. C. and Jones, B. R. (1972) Clinical trial of topical disodium cromoglycate in vernal kerato-conjunctivitis. *Clin. Allergy*, **2**, 99.

18. Easty, D. L. (1977) *Topical Sodium Cromoglycate in Vernal Kerato-conjunctivitis.* Proceedings XI European Congress of Allergology and Clinical Immunology, Prague, September.

CHAPTER 10

Allergic Reaction to Insect Bites and Stings

THE STINGING INSECTS are responsible for about 5 to 6 deaths a year in the United Kingdom, and 40 to 50 in the United States.[2,3,4] The true incidence of insect stings is unknown but must be considerable.

The reactions caused by stinging insects range from a mild local inflammatory change associated with swelling, pain and erythema and lasting for a number of hours, to severe local response with considerable and diffuse oedema which often persists for some days. This is especially so following a wasp sting which may carry bacteria and cause cellulitis.[5,6] Generalised reactions may occur within a few minutes after a sting but may also be delayed for 24 hours or more. Clinical features may consist of angioedema, urticaria, vomiting, acute bronchospasm and occasionally acute circulatory failure. Multiple stings may cause severe toxic reactions. It has been suggested that during a sting about 0·05 ml of venom is injected into the skin.[7]

Fleas (dog, cat) and mites typically cause papular urticaria which often gives a biphasic response. Within minutes of the bite an immediate reaction occurs to be followed in 24 to 48 hours by a delayed sensitivity resulting in an indurated papule. Such papules can persist for many weeks or even months. If the papules are examined histologically, they can mimic various conditions, e.g. lymphoma.

There exists well over a million species of insects but relatively few are responsible for untoward reactions in the human.[1] Most insects bite in order to obtain nourishment. The few that sting do so most probably in self-defence.

Biting insects

The most commonly encountered are horse flies, gnats and midges, mosquitoes, harvest mites and fleas. The female horse fly, because of strong sucking pads, often cause large bites which bleed. Gnats, midges and mosquitoes inflict multiple bites which cause severe itching. The most severe local reactions from a mosquito bite in the United Kingdom are caused by *Theobaldia annulata* species recognised easily by its white and black bands on the legs. Harvest mites, as the name suggests (watch out for insect with six legs, red in colour and about 0·2–0·5 mm in length) are found in fields during the summer and early autumn days.

They bite exposed parts of the body (legs, arms and thighs) and cause minor localised reactions in non-allergic individuals. Hypersensitive subjects not uncommonly develop severe local reactions such as the formation of vesicles or even blisters.

Stinging insects

There are at least tens of thousands of species of Hymenoptera but only four families cause allergic reactions in men: honey bees, hornets, wasps and bumble-bees.

Venoms of insects, bees and wasps contain many antigens some of which can be isolated from the saliva, the venom itself, or from the body of the insect. There is some evidence that reactions such as swelling and pain are due to the release of histamine, acetylcholine, kinins, serotonin and other similar mediators. The generalised anaphylactic responses are most likely mediated by IgE and necessarily do not occur in an individual who is atopic or was born into an atopic family.[8,9]

In general, most serious reactions follow repeated minor episodes but in 5 to 8 per cent of subjects an initial exposure may result in severe symptoms. The most severe reactions occur within a short period following a sting, but occasionally may be delayed for some hours. The Hymenoptera venoms contain many pharmacologically active substances such as histamine, mellitin, phospholipase A and B, hyaluronidase, allergens B and C, apamin and lecithinase.[10–12]

If an allergic reaction occurs following a sting there will be a persistent rise of IgE antibody levels reaching the maximum in about 14 to 21 days. Interestingly if the patients are tested with a number of specific venoms immediate Type I reactions and rise of serum IgE can be either to one or two of the venoms only but not to venoms of other insects.[13,14] It is important to bear this in mind when immunotherapy is being considered.

Diagnosis

Although a positive history of stinging is often obvious, identification of the insect with the exception of the honey bee which leaves its sting behind can be very difficult. Skin sensitivity tests in order to identify if the child is at risk from reactions are misleading. They are of value in predicting the lowest dilution of extract to be used for hyposensitisation in a child who previously has had a generalised reaction. Demonstration of specific IgE in serum for bee venom are available and can be easily performed by the radioallergosorbent test (RAST), but it is too early to comment on the practical significance of a positive finding. Similarly, studies of the release of histamine by leucocytes by insect sensitive subjects may offer better guidance in identifying individuals at risk from severe reactions.[15-21]

Treatment

Insect bites

The majority of insect bites can be successfully managed by a topical application of calamine lotion, a corticosteroid or antihistamine cream or ointment. It is worth remembering that bites caused by the horse-fly may become infected—if so, an antibiotic should be given.

Insect stings

Bee stings should be removed immediately with tweezers or scraped out with the blade of a knife. Attempts to remove a sting with the fingers usually results in it being pushed deeper into the skin and should be avoided. A sting inside the mouth should be removed if possible, but not much time spent on a search for it because not uncommonly severe oedema may quickly develop and cause breathing and swallowing difficulties. In such situations an immediate injection of 0·2–0·5 ml of adrenaline 1:1000 should be given s.c. If available hydrocortisone hemisuccinate 200 mg should be given i.v. or i.m. and the child admitted to the nearest hospital. If signs of shock appear, small doses of 1:1000 adrenaline can be administered every 15 to 20 minutes and large i.v. doses of hydrocortisone. If massive angioedema occurs plasma or plasma expanders are required to restore blood volume and cardiac output. The value of applying a tourniquet to a limb about the sting site remains undecided.[22] Occasionally a child is stung in the eye. If so, topical and systemic corticosteroids should be used, antihistamines and antibiotics as discussed above. Attempts at removal of the sting should be discouraged since little damage can be done to the eye—the inert sting can be left safely and indefinitely in the cornea or anterior chamber without causing any eye problems.[23]

Long-term management

To witness a generalised insect sting reaction is a frightening experience for the child and his family. Common sense advice should be offered as how to minimise the exposure to the offending insects, e.g. white clothing during the summer months reduces attraction, the wearing of proper shoes when at play, the avoidance of parks and bright flowers and the use of insecticides when indoors, keeping windows (car as well) closed and above all, not to panic when an insect is within reach but to stand still or slowly move away. The parents should keep oral and intramuscular antihistamines at home. An adrenaline kit is a useful standby.

The use of hyposensitisation should be considered if the child has had severe local or general reactions. A skin test is performed first with the lowest dilution of the extract which will give a positive reaction. This is the starting dose—usually 0·02–0·05 ml concentration. Subsequently, weekly doses are given at increasing concentrations up to 1:10 and a dose of 0·5 ml. In order to maintain a high level of protection monthly, two monthly or three monthly injections should be continued indefinitely.

There is evidence that 95 per cent of those who continue with such a scheme experience fewer reactions when re-stung. In a 20-year-old follow up study of 400 patients who had 3 years of hyposensitisation with the whole body extract on a maintenance dose equivalent to one or more stings, only 6 per cent developed systemic symptoms of some degree following stings.[28] Better results appear to be obtained if higher and prolonged (more than 3 years) extracts can be employed.[14,24,25,28,29] Superior results are obtained when pure insect venoms are used.[26,27] However, although honey bee venom is easily extracted, the pure preparation of other insect venom extracts remains difficult.

References

1. Imms, A. D. (1971) *Insect Natural History*. 3rd ed. p. 2. London: Collins.
2. Barnard, J. H. (1973) Studies of 400 Hymenoptera sting deaths in the United States. *J. Allergy Clin. Immunol.*, **52**, 259.
3. Reid, H. A. (1976) Adder bites in Britain. *Br. med. J.*, **II**, 153.
4. Barr, S. E. (1971) Allergy to Hymenoptera stings—Review of the world literature, 1953–70. *Annls Allergy*, **29**, 49.
5. Frazier, C. A. (1969) *Insect Allergy*. St. Louis: Warren H. Green.
6. Bucherl, W. and Buckley, E. (1971) Venomous Animals and their Venoms. Vol. 2, p. 3. Illinois: Charles C. Thomas.
7. Barr, S. E. (1974) Allergy to Hymenoptera stings. *J. Am. med. Ass.*, **228**, 718.
8. Settipane, G. A., Newstead, G. J. and Boyd, G. K. (1972) Frequency of Hymenoptera allergy in an atopic and normal population. *J. Allergy Clin. Immunol.*, **50**, 146.
9. Shulman, S. (1969) Insect allergy. Biochemical and immunological analysis of the antigens. *Progr. Allergy*, **12**, 246.
10. Hoffman, D. R., Shipman, W. H. and Babin, D. (1977) Allergens in bee venom—II. Two new high molecular weight allergenic specificities. *J. Allergy Clin. Immunol.*, **59**, 147.
11. King, T. P., Sobotka, A. K., Kochoumian, L. and Lichtenstein, L. M. (1976) Allergens of honey bee venom. *Archs Biochem. Biophys.*, **172**, 661.
12. Hoffman, D. R. (1977) Allergens in bee venom—III. Identification of allergen B of bee venom as an acid phosphatase. *J. Allergy Clin. Immunol.*, **59**, 364.

13. Reisman, R. E., Wypych, J. I., Yeagle, N. and Arbesman, C. E. (1974) Stinging insect hypersensitivity—III. Detection and clinical significance of IgE antibodies to insect venom in man. *J. Allergy Clin. Immunol.*, **53**, 110.
14. Reisman, R. E. and Arbesman, C. E. (1975) Stinging insect allergy. Current concepts and problems. *Pediatr. Clin. N. Am.*, **22**, 185.
15. Sobotka, A. K., Valentine, M. D., Benton, A. W. and Lichtenstein, L. M. (1974) Allergy to insect stings—I. Diagnosis of IgE mediated Hymenoptera sensitivity by venom induced histamine release. *J. Allergy and Clin. Immunol.*, **53**, 170.
16. Hoffman, D. R. (1977) Allergens in Hymenoptera venoms—IV. Comparison of venom and venom sac extracts. *J. Allergy Clin. Immunol.*, **59**, 367.
17. Yocum, M. W., Johnstone, D. E. and Condemi, J. J. (1973) Leucocyte histamine release in Hymenoptera allergic patients. *J. Allergy Clin. Immunol.*, **52**, 265.
18. Mackler, B. F., Russell, A. S. and Kreil, G. (1972) Allergenic and biological activities of melittin from honey bee venom. *Clin. Allergy*, **2**, 317.
19. Brenton, H. S. and Brown, H. (1965) Studies on the Hymenoptera—I. Skin reactions of normal persons to the honey bee (*Apis mellifera*) extract. *J. Allergy*, **36**, 315.
20. Schwartz, H. J. (1965) Skin sensitivity in insect allergy. *J. Am. med. Ass.*, **194**, 703.
21. Müller, U., Spiess, J. and Roth, A. (1977) Serological investigations in Hymenoptera sting allergy: IgE and haemagglutinating antibodies against bee venom in patients with bee sting allergy, bee keepers and non-allergic blood-donors. *Clin. Allergy*, **7**, 147.
22. Frazier, C. A. (1976) Insect stings—a medical emergency. *J. Am. med. Ass.*, **235**, 2410.
23. Gilboa, M., Gdal-on, M. and Zonis, S. (1977) Bee and wasp stings of the eye. Retained intralenticular wasp sting: a case report. *Br. J. Ophthalmol.*, **61**, 662.
24. Lessof, M. H., Sobotka, A. K. and Lichtenstein, L. M. (1976) Protection against anaphylaxis in Hymenoptera-sensitive patients by passive immunisation. *J. Allergy Clin. Immunol.*, **57**, 246.
25. Lichtenstein, L. M., Valentine, M. D. and Sobotka, A. K. (1974) A case for venous treatment in anaphylactic sensitivity to Hymenoptera sting. *New Eng. Med. J.*, **290**, 1223.
26. Franklin, R. and Baer, H. (1975) Comparison of honey bee venoms and their components from various sources. *J. Allergy Clin. Immunol.*, **55**, 285.
27. Busse, W. W., Reed, C. E. and Lichtenstein, L. M. (1975) Immunotherapy in bee-sting anaphylaxis. Use of honey bee venom. *J. Am. med. Ass.*, **231**, 1154.
28. Mueller, H. L. (1975) Stinging-insect hypersensitivity: a 20 year study of immunologic treatment. *Pediatrics*, **55**, 4.
29. Mueller, H. L. (1977) Maintenance of protection in patients treated for stinging insect hypersensitivity: a booster injection program. *Pediatrics*, **59**, 773.

CHAPTER 11

Drug Allergy

ALTHOUGH ADVERSE REACTIONS to drugs have been recognised for centuries, it is barely 25 years since registries have been set up for the purpose of collecting information of suspected toxic effects of drug treatment. Such an approach is of necessity incomplete because it is impossible to know precisely how many individuals actually take drugs, singly or in combination, and more importantly it is difficult to be sure at times that an adverse reaction has occurred. The World Health Organisation survey estimated that per 10,000 treated patients there were 1–4 reactions and 0·15–0·2 deaths.[28] About 10 per cent of hospital patients are known to develop some drug reaction, but since many patients receive other drugs simultaneously, e.g. five in the United Kingdom and nine in the hospitals of the United States, it can be almost impossible to detect the real culprit.

Documentation of adverse reactions to drugs outside hospital is scanty. It has been estimated that about 30 per cent of patients discharged from medical wards in a New Zealand hospital subsequently developed drug reactions and every fortieth patient seen by a General Practitioner does so because of side-effects of drugs which he is taking. The opportunities of developing reactions to drugs are enormous. An average household in the United Kingdom has at least three drug containers of which a not insignificant proportion is formed by antibiotics.[1-7]

In general allergic children do not develop reactions to drugs more often than normal children although some studies suggest that sensitivity to penicillin and aspirin products is more common.[8-11] In an extensive study, it was found that 5 per cent of patients developed allergic reactions (conjunctivitis, skin rashes, fever) and if a second course was needed the prevalence of allergic reactions rose to 11·1 per cent. In those who experienced initial reactions the incidence increased to 16·2 per cent. Moreover, if the same agent caused reactions initially, and the patients were given the same drug again, the rate rose to 68·8 per cent.[31]

A useful practical classification of adverse drug reactions is comprised of two broad categories:

a. reactions which can occur in any normal child because the drug happens to have side-effects; overdosage is given leading to widespread toxic manifestations; or when combined with another agent alters its own, or the other agent's pharmacologic actions;

b. reactions which can occur in a sensitive child because of genetic or metabolic factors causing immunological reactions, idiosyncrasy or intolerance (Table 11.1).

Table 11.1   Types of drug reactions

1. *Reactions in a normal child:*
   a. Side-effect
   b. Over-dosage
   c. Drug interactions

2. *Reactions in a sensitive child:*
   a. Allergy:
   Type I reaction, e.g. anaphylactic shock, urticaria.
   Type II reaction, e.g. thrombocytopoenic purpura, haemolytic anaemia.
   Type III reaction, e.g. vasculitis, serum sickness, skin rash, kidney lesions, anaphylactoid purpura.
   Type IV reaction, e.g. fixed drug eruptions.

   b. Intolerance
   c. Idiosyncrasy

Immunological aspects

Allergic drug reactions may involve Types I–IV mechanisms.[23] Drugs, in general, have a low molecular weight and in order to elicit an immunological reaction have to be coupled to a larger molecule such as a protein. The substance so coupled is known as a hapten and the formed antigen as a conjugate. The binding is often irreversible in contrast to the reversible affinity many drugs have to plasma proteins. It follows that before any chemical agent is capable of initiating an immune response the subject must have been previously exposed to the agent or a related compound which then forms a stable conjugate with a protein carrier. The sensitisation interval can vary, i.e. can occur rapidly during the first few days of the drug therapy and allergic manifestations can be provoked during the actual treatment course or may take 7 to 14 days or so. Haptens do not elicit immune responses even in a very sensitive child. However, there is evidence that some molecules which show minimal coupling with proteins may cause allergic reactions. The mechanism in these situations is unclear. With some agents, e.g. penicillin, Type I immediate skin reactions and a rise in specific IgE antibodies can be demonstrated to penicilloyl polylysine. This however, does not imply that the symptoms are due to the agent but confirms that the individual has been immunised to it. Relatively good correlation is obtained between skin sensitivity testing and serum IgE to penicilloyl polylysine or enzyme penicillin. In general, the correlation between skin tests and drug allergy varies between 10 and 90 per cent. Occasionally urticarial responses occur 6 to 48 hours after the administration of a drug and may be associated with a rise in IgE serum levels.[12–19,22,24]

Similarly haemagglutinating antibodies of the class IgM and IgG can be demonstrated in many subjects who have not been exposed to a particular drug for many years. It is possible that the IgE antibody formation may have resulted from stimulation by traces of penicillin in foods and other dairy products.

Some children may develop serum sickness type of reactions which closely resemble responses to a serum used in passive immunisation. In this type of reaction antibodies of the class IgG or IgM react with an antigenic component of a cell or hapten which has been associated with the cell. Complement is involved and the cell destroyed.[20,23]

The skin contact hypersensitivity and the tuberculin response are classical examples of Type IV (delayed) hypersensitivity reactions. Some drugs, e.g. penicillin, may occasionally give rise to such a reaction around the site where the agent has been injected. Antibodies responsible for the immediate (skin sensitivity) reactions are absent but a significant rise of the IgM class can be observed. It has also been suggested that these drug responses may involve non-immunological mechanisms.[9,13,21–23]

Clinical presentations of adverse drug reactions

Anaphylactic reaction (coined by Portier and Richet—opposite of phylaxis or protection)[25]

Many substances and drugs can be responsible for anaphylactic reactions but the most frequently encountered in children are agents from foods such as cow's milk, egg, fish, etc., antibiotics, e.g. penicillin and its derivatives, chloramphenicol, cephalosporins, streptomycin and tetracycline; foreign sera, vaccines; and extracts of allergens; local anaesthetic agents; aspirins and similar compounds; diagnostic contract media and anticonvulsants, e.g. phenytoin.[26]

Between 1966 and 1975, the Committee on Safety of Medicines (U.K.) received reports of 140 anaphylactic reactions to drugs of which 41 were directly responsible for death. Autopsy findings consist of widespread oedema especially involving the upper respiratory tract and lungs and tissue oesinophilia at times most striking in the lungs and the liver.[27,29,30]

The symptoms arise within seconds or minutes after exposure to the agent after an initial 2 to 5 day interval following the first dose. The earlier clinical manifestations occur after drug taking, the more severe they become.

The diagnosis is straightforward although occasionally confusion may arise in distinguishing early features of anaphylaxis from urticaria and hereditary angioedema.

Clinical features consist of a rapid onset of erythematous and urticarial rash which may be accompanied by respiratory distress and generalised constitutional upset consisting of sweating, chest and abdominal cramps, vomiting and diarrhoea often containing blood and leading to upper airway obstruction and shock. Convulsions and loss of consciousness occur relatively late.

Treatment

Speed is essential

Adrenaline 1:1000 solution should be given immediately i.v. (0.01 ml/kg) and repeated within 15 minutes.

Acute respiratory distress and airway obstruction should be treated by i.v. administration of aminophylline (5 mg/kg), slowly, i.e. 5 to 10 minutes.

Administration of an antihistamine agent given i.v. is helpful in reducing oedema, itching and the rash.

Although corticosteroids are often used initially, it should be remembered that they exert their maximum effect in 2 to 6 hours. Thus, they should be given immediately after the initial treatment as described above, because of their powerful anti-inflammatory action. Intravenous infusion of loading and maintenance doses of hydrocortisone (10 mg/kg) should be commenced and administered for the next 6 to 24 hours.

Vital supportive measures

Ensure adequate airway.

Give oxygen by face mask. Beware of hypoxia. If there is evidence of laryngeal obstruction from oedema, endotracheal intubation should be performed forthwith and assisted ventilation commenced. Some children become hypovolaemic. It is essential to correct such a deficit with saline and plasma infusions. If the child remains hypotensive—infuse continuously metaraminol bitartrate 0.3 mg/kg to maintain adequate tissue perfusion. Observe the child's progress very carefully for 2 to 3 days as late relapse may happen.

It is useful to monitor ECG changes as a guide to recovery, inversion of T wave or elevation of ST segment persists for a number of days, but remember sometimes abnormal ECG changes are absent.

Following recovery from an anaphylactic shock a detailed investigation of the causative drug should be made and the parents issued with a full list of related compounds which may cause reactions. It should be insisted that any future drugs should be given orally as there is some evidence that the oral route is associated with a lower incidence of hypersensitivity than any other. The wearing of a medallion or emblem stating that the child experienced severe anaphylactic reaction has much to commend it and should be strongly encouraged.

Skin manifestations

There is no known drug which causes a specific skin rash. Any rash may occur and stimulate bacterial, viral or other infections. Drugs commonly giving rise to skin manifestations in children are: antibiotics such as penicillin, streptomycin and neomycin, antihistamines and barbiturates, sulphonamides and derivatives, phenytoin and derivatives and certain parabens; sera and cytotoxic agents. Histological examination of the skin shows a perivascular infiltrate with eosinophils and damage to the vessel walls.

Toxic erythema

The appearance of a morbiliform-like rash in a child who has had measles strongly suggests reaction. When in doubt it is worth excluding drug allergy by performing virus studies—the number of children who have been credited with 'measles' twice or even three times in their short lives is not an uncommon observation!

Nevertheless, the eruption may be papular or vesicular and even bullous. Agents applied directly to the skin are commonly responsible for episodes of contact dermatitis. The most common are antibiotics such as neomycin, antihistamines, parabens (preservatives) and local anaesthetic agents. It should also be remembered that some agents applied to the skin may cause reaction following exposure to sun, e.g. sun-tan lotions, medicated soaps, etc.

Erythema multiforme (Stevens–Johnson syndrome)

An acute papular and erythematous rash occurs and quickly becomes vesicular leading to the formation of bullae. There is an associated involvement of mucous membranes of the mouth and eyes and/or genital tract. Constitutional symptoms are often present. The most commonly involved drugs are barbiturates and long-acting sulphonamides. The condition continues waxing and waning for between 7 and 28 days and is responsible for mortality of 5 to 10 per cent.[37] Toxic epidermal necrolysis (Lyell's Syndrome) although most commonly caused by a specific phage type staphylococcal skin infection has been associated with drug treatment, e.g. antibiotics, sulphonamides, phenytoin, etc. There is generalised erythematous rash leading to the formation of bullae and desquamation. Death may result from overwhelming infection. Recovery is usually rapid and complete. Management consists of nursing the child as for second-degree burns (sterile room, prevention of staphylococcal and streptococcal infections, maintenance of protein and electrolyte balance and renal function—i.v. infusions of hydrocortisone 5 mg/kg).

Erythema nodosum

There occurs symmetrical bilateral erythematous and nodular rash over the anterior aspects of legs. Not uncommonly the child complains of joint pains and has a low grade fever. The agents most commonly involved are antibiotics; sulphonamides and salicylates and related compounds.

Fixed drug eruption

A round swelling which may become vesicular, haemorrhagic and pruritic, appears at the injection site. It may persist for two or more weeks after a drug has been discontinued and leave behind an area of pigmentation. The common agents involved are antibiotics, sulphonamides, hypnotics and quinidine.

Allergic vasculitis

The rash is predominantly macular or macular-papular and associated with a degree of pruritus, and purpura occasionally may be associated with oedema and urticaria. The classical Schonlein–Henoch Syndrome distribution over the extremities and buttocks may occur. If small blood vessels of the gastro-intestinal tract and kidneys are involved there will be episodes of abdominal pain, blood in stools and urine. The skin eruptions usually persist for one or more weeks and may recur. The most commonly implicated drugs are salicylates and antibiotics.[44]

Acute cutaneous angiitis

Dependent parts of the body and those subjected to external pressure are affected. Large areas of purpura or bruising are seen. The lesions involve the veins causing thrombosis. Associated lesions such as polyarteritis nodosa and drug induced lupus erythematosus are rarely seen in children. Drugs known to involve children are some anti-convulsants, e.g. phenytoin, antibiotics, e.g. penicillin, streptomycin, sulphonamides and chlorpromazine.[32–35,38]

Serum sickness

Serum sickness caused by drug allergy occurs a few days after a drug has been administered. The child develops a generalised urticarial eruption which may be erythematous, joint swelling, lymphadenopathy and pyrexia. There may be bronchospasm and evidence of hepatitis. The clinical features persist for from 4 to 14 days but may be prolonged if a long-acting drug was used, e.g. sulphonamide. Apart from foreign sera, agents which most commonly cause serum sickness are: antibiotics especially penicillin and streptomycin and anticonvulsants, e.g. phenytoin, barbiturates.[36] Treatment consists of stopping all drugs immediately, administration of an antihistamine, e.g. diphenhydramine 4 mg/kg to combat itching and urticaria and prednisolone 2 mg/kg daily for arthralgia and pyrexia for a number of days.

Blood

Three effects have been described following therapy: haemolytic anaemia due to large doses of penicillin, agranulocytoses due to chloramphenicol and sulphonamides and thrombocytopenia (with pyrexia and joint swelling) following the administration of sulphonamides, chlorothiazide, frusemide, quinine and its analogues.[38]

Kidneys

The renal tract may be involved as part of serum sickness or lupus erythematosus hypersensitivity reactions and directly as interstitial nephritis associated with the administration of analgesics and acute glomerulonephritis due to antibiotics, sulphonamides, gold salts, troxidone, etc. Histologically there is evidence of tubular degeneration and glomerulocapillary necrosis.[40]

Lungs

Acute bronchospasm may occur as part of an anaphylactic reaction or be caused directly by drugs. Pulmonary changes may consist of widespread transient infiltrates, hilar gland enlargement and plural involvement. The features may persist for many weeks. The most commonly implicated agents are penicillin and its derivatives, sulphonamides, nitrofurantoin and methotrexate.[41,42]

Eyes

Type I reactions may be caused by local administration of antibiotics and will be characterised by oedema of the conjunctiva and the lids. The eyes may be involved in the Stevens–Johnson Syndrome and occasionally as a part of serum sickness. Contact dermatitis may be caused by antibiotics, atropine and local ointments.[39,42,43]

Diagnosis

The most important aspect is a history of previous reaction to an identical drug or a similar compound. Blood examination may show eosinophilia and a low serum complement. Skin sensitivity tests are of most value in suspected penicillin allergy but should be carried out with great caution as anaphylactic reactions may occur.[45,46] They are unhelpful in other drug allergies. The use of the skin window technique is difficult in practice and the results are unreliable. Similarly the Prausnitz-Küstner test (transfer of the patient's serum to the skin of normal recipient) is too risky.

In vitro tests

The most useful investigation in detecting penicillin allergy is by the use of the radioallergosorbent test (RAST) which correlates well with the skin tests and clinical history.[19,47] There is a number of other specialised tests which may be helpful in the diagnosis of drug allergies.[52,53] The basophil degranulation test (direct and indirect) was designed to demonstrate anaphylactic reagenic antibodies in sera of penicillin allergic subjects. However, the test has not met with general approval.[48] The passive sensitisation tests using either human leucocytes or human and monkey lungs have been found useful but of necessity are expensive, very technical and thus unlikely to be widely available.[49] The lymphocyte transformation method was developed to test the delayed type of drug reactions but was found to be relatively insensitive.[50,51]

Preventive measures

Great caution should be exercised in prescribing drugs in children. The parents should be fully aware of which drugs to avoid and as few as possible used. On rare occasions hyposensitisation may be attempted if clinically indicated. It is almost entirely confined to penicillin allergy and consists in administering increasing doses of penicillin over a period of time starting with 1 unit/ml and rapidly increasing until 1 mega unit is given s.c. without any adverse effects. A child who has had a severe drug reaction should carry a warning card at all times.

References

1. Leach, R. H. and White, P. L. (1978) Use and wastage of prescribed medicines in the home. *J. R. Col. gen. Pract.*, **28**, 33, 86.
2. Dunlop, D. (1965) Use and abuse of drugs. *Br. med. J.*, **II**, 437.
3. Hurwitz, N. and Wade, O. L. (1969) Intensive hospital monitoring of adverse reactions to drugs. *Br. med. J.*, **I**, 531.

4. Boston Collaborative Drug Surveillance Program (1972) *Pediatr. Clin. N. Am.*, **19**, 117.
5. Levy, M., Nir, I. and Superstine, E. (1974) Antimicrobial therapy in patients hospitalised in a medical ward. *Israel J. med. Sci.*, **II**, 322.
6. Kellaway, G. S. and McCrae, E. (1975) Non-compliance and errors of drug administration in patients discharged from acute medical wards. *N.Z. med. J.*, **78**, 525.
7. Mulroy, R. (1973) Iatrogenic disease in general practice: Its incidence and effects. *Brit. med. J.*, **II**, 407.
8. Steinber, R. H. and Levine, B. (1973) Prevalence of allergic diseases, pencillin hypersensitivity and aeroallergen hypersensitivity in various populations. Abstract 46. *Am. Acad. Allergy*, **5**, 100.
9. Levine, B. (1968) Immunochemical mechanism of drug allergy. In: *Textbook of Immunopathology*. Ed. by Miescher, P. A. and Muller-Eberhard, H. J., Vol. 1, p. 271. New York: Graham-Stratton.
10. Rosh, M. S. and Shinefield, H. R. (1968) Penicillin antibodies in children. *Pediatrics*, **42**, 342.
11. Giraldo, B., Blumenthal, M. N. and Spink, W. W. (1969) Aspirin intolerance and asthma. *Ann. intern. Med.*, **71**, 479.
12. De Weck, A. L. (1971) Drug reactions. In: *Immunological Diseases*. Ed. by Samter, M., 2nd ed., pp. 415–440. Boston: Little Brown.
13. Juhlin, L. and Wide, L. (1972) IgE antibodies and penicillin allergy. In: *Mechanisms in Drug Allergy*. Ed. by Dash, C. H. and Jones, H. E. R., pp. 139–147. Glaxo Symposium Series. Edinburgh: Churchill Livingstone.
14. Levine, B. (1966) Immunologic mechanisms of penicillin allergy. *New Eng. Med. J.*, **275**, 1115.
15. Stember, R. H. and Levine, B. B. (1972) Frequency of skin reactivity to penicillin haptens in patients without histories of penicillin allergy. *J. Allergy Clin. Immunol.*, **49**, 96.
16. Carr, E. A. and Aste, G. A. (1961) Recent laboratory studies and clinical observations on hypersensitivity to drugs and use of drugs in allergy. *A. rev. Pharmac.*, **1**, 105.
17. Shmunes, E. (1977) Occult penicillin exposure reaction. *Ann. Allergy*, **39**, 186.
18. Prince, H. E. (1977) Aspirin and cross reactivity (editorial). *Annls Allergy*, **39**, 47.
19. Kraft, D., Roth, A., Mischer, P., Pilcher, H. and Ebner, H. (1977) Specific and total serum IgE measurements in the diagnosis of penicillin allergy. A long-term follow-up study. *Clin. Allergy*, **7**, 21.
20. Arbesman, C. E. and Reisman, R. E. (1971) Serum sickness and human anaphylaxis. In: *Immunological Diseases*. Ed. by Samter, M., 2nd ed., pp. 405–414. Boston: Little Brown.
21. Marsh, D. G., Hsu, S. H. and Bias, W. B. (1973) The genetic basis for atopic allergy in man. *J. Allergy Clin. Immunol.*, **51**, 80.
22. Bazaral, M., Orgel, H. A. and Hamburger, R. N. (1974) Genetics of IgE and allergy. Serum IgE levels in twins. *J. Allergy Clin. Immunol.*, **54**, 288.
23. Acroyd, J. F. (1975) Immunological mechanisms in drug hypersensitivity. In: *Clinical Aspects of Immunology*. Ed. by Gell, P. G. H., Coomb, R. R. A. and Lachmann, P. J., 3rd ed., pp. 913–952. Oxford: Blackwell Scientific.
24. Müller, U., Morrell, A. and Hoigne, R. (1973) IgE in allergic drug reactions. *Int. Archs. Allergy appl. Immunol.*, **44**, 667.
25. Portier, P. and Richet, C. (1902) De d'action anaphylactique de certains venins. *C. Soc. Biol.*, **54**, 170.
26. Siegel, S. C. and Heimlich, E. M. (1962) Anaphylaxis. *Pediatr. Clin. N. Am.*, **9**, 29.
27. Committee on Safety of Medicines (1977) Personal communication.
28. Idsoe, O. (1968) *Bulletin World Health Organization*, **38**, 159.
29. Sparks, R. P. (1971) Fatal anaphylaxis due to oral penicillin. *Am. J. clin. Pathol.*, **56**, 407.
30. Rosenthal, A. (1958) Follow-up study of fatal penicillin reactions. *J. Am. med. Ass.*, **167**, 1118.

31. Dowling, H. F., Hirsh, H. L. and Lepper, M. H. (1946) Toxic reactions accompanying second courses of sulphonamides in patients developing toxic reactions during a previous course. *Ann. intern. Med.*, **24**, 629.
32. Copeman, P. W. M. and Ryan, T. J. (1970) The problems of classification of cutaneous angiitis with reference to histopathology and pathogenesis. *Br. J. Dermatol.* Suppl. 5, **82**, 26.
33. Savin, J. A. (1970) Current causes of fixed drug eruptions. *Br. J. Dermatol.*, **83**, 546.
34. Bass, J. W., Crowley, D. M., Steele, R. W., Young, F. S. H. and Harden, L. B. (1973) Adverse effects of orally administered ampicillin. *J. Pediatr.*, **83**, 106.
35. Schneider, C. H. (1974) Specific reactions to specific drugs: penicillin. In: *Allergology.* Ed. by Yamamura, Y., pp. 437–440. Amsterdam: Excerpta Medica.
36. Bruinsma, W. (1973) A Guide to Drug Eruptions. Amsterdam: Excerpta Medica.
37. Almeyda, J. and Levantine, A. (1972) Cutaneous reactions to barbiturates, chloral hydrate and its derivatives. *Br. J. Dermatol.*, **86**, 313.
38. Meyler, L. and Herxheimer, A. (Eds.) (1972) *Side-effects of Drugs.* Amsterdam: Excerpta Medica.
39. Mushin, A. S. (1972) Ocular damage by drugs in children. *Adverse Drug Reaction Bull.*, **36**, 112.
40. Schrier, R. W., Bulger, R. T. and Van Arsdel, P. P. (1966) Nephropathy associated with penicillin and homologues. *Archs. intern. Med.*, **64**, 116.
41. Nichlaus, T. M. and Snyder, A. B. (1968) Nitrofuradantin pulmonary reaction. *Archs. intern. Med.*, **121**, 151.
42. Turner-Warwick, M., Assem, E. S. K. and Lockwood, M. (1976) Crypto genic pulmonary eosinophilia. *Clin. Allergy*, **6**, 135.
43. Crews, S. J. (1977) Ocular adverse reactions to drugs. *The Practitioner*, **219**, 72.
44. Giangiocomo, J. and Tsai, C. C. (1977) Dermal and glomerular deposition of IgA in anaphylactoid purpura. *Am. J. Dis. Child.*, **131**, 981.
45. Finke, S. R., Grieco, M. H., Connell, J. T., Smith, E. C. and Serman, W. B. (1965) Results of comparative skin tests with penicilloyl-polylysine and penicillin in patients with penicillin allergy. *Am. J. Med.*, **38**, 71.
46. Idsoe, O., Guthe, T., Willcox, R. R. and De Weck, A. L. (1968) Nature and extent of penicillin side-reactions, with particular reference to fatalities from anaphylactic shock. *Bull. Wld. Hlth. Org.*, **38**, 159.
47. Kraft, D. and Wide, L. (1976) Clinical patterns and results of radioallergosorbent test (RAST) and skin tests in penicillin allergy. *Br. J. Dermatol.*, **94**, 593.
48. Hubscher, T., Watson, J. I. and Goodfried, L. (1970) Target cells of human ragweed-binding antibodies in monkey skin. *J. Immunol.*, **104**, 1196.
49. Assem, E. S. K. and Schild, H. O. (1968) Detection of allergy to penicillin and other antigens by in vitro passive sensitisation and histamine release from human and monkey lung. *Br. med. J.*, **III**, 272.
50. Vischer, T. L. (1966) Lymphocyte cultures in drug hypersensitivity. *Lancet*, **II**, 467.
51. Reichenberger, M. and Heitmann, H. J. (1969) Lymphocyte transformation in patients allergic to ampicillin and tetracyline. *Lancet*, **II**, 491.
52. Voss, H. E., Redmond, A. P. and Levine, B. B. (1966) Clinical detection of the potential allergic reactor to penicillin by immunologic tests. *J. Am. med. Ass.*, **196**, 679.
53. Saurat, J. H., Burtin, C. B., Soubrane, C. B. and Paupe, J. R. (1973) Cell mediated hypersensitivity in skin reactions to drugs (except contact dermatitis). *Clin. Allergy.*, **3**, 427.

CHAPTER 12

Allergy and Cystic Fibrosis

THERE IS SOME evidence suggesting that many children with cystic fibrosis (CF) are also atopic subjects (in one study 15 per cent) and that the immunological responses produced may cause the characteristic pathological features seen in CF, i.e. progressive lung damage and pancreatic or even hepatic involvement.[1-4] However, the importance of allergic factors in the pathogenesis of CF is far from clear.

Children with CF often demonstrate Type I immediate skin hypersensitivity reactions to various allergens such as house dust, diary products and meats, animal epithelia and fungi. It is most unusual to observe positive hypersensitivity reactions to *D. pteronyssinus* and grass pollens in a CF child or to obtain a positive history of atopic dermatitis. About 50 per cent of CF children give positive reactions to *A. fumigatus* in comparison to 10 to 20 per cent of individuals with bronchial asthma.[5-8] The total and specific serum IgE levels are often considerably elevated. A suggestion has been made that the degree of rise may be related to the severity of the disease.[5,9,11] Some children may also show rises of IgG 4 levels—possibly representing an antibody response to bacterial infections.[10]

There are also indications that there may exist a defect in the synthesis of secretory IgA and this may explain the presence of immune complexes in many organs of CF children. Indeed the development of allergy may be related to transient IgA deficiency.[12-14]

Although the recent studies are of considerable interest and importance, it is worth pointing out that many of the observations described may represent secondary phenomena of the complications which are common in this relatively rapid and progressive disease.

References

1. Van Metre, T. E., Cooke, R., Gibson, L. E. and Winkelwerder, W. L. (1960) Evidence of allergy in patients with cystic fibrosis. *J. Allergy*, **31**, 141.
2. Schwarchman, H., Kulczycki, L. L., Mueller, H. L. (1962) Nasal polyposis in patients with cystic fibrosis. *Pediatrics*, **30**, 389.
3. Yohe, R. M. (1972) Allergy in patients with cystic fibrosis. *Annls Allergy*, **30**, 627.

4. Wallwork, J. C., Brenchley, P., McCarthy, J., Allan, J. D., Moss, A. D., Ward, A. M., Holzel, A., Williams, R. F. and McFarlane, H. (1974) Some aspects of immunity in patients with cystic fibrosis. *Clin. exp. Immunol.*, **18**, 303.
5. Allan, J. D., Moss, A. D., Wallwork, J. C. and McFarlane, H. (1975) Immediate hypersensitivity in patients with cystic fibrosis. *Clin. Allergy*, **5**, 255.
6. Mearns, M., Longbottom, J. L. and Batten, J. C. (1967) Precipitating antibodies to *Aspergillus fumigatus* in cystic fibrosis. *Lancet*, **I**, 538.
7. McCarthy, D. S., Pepys, J. and Batten, J. C. (1969) Hypersensitivity to fungi in cystic fibrosis. *Proc. 5th Int. Cystic Fibrosis Conf.*
8. Warren, C. P. W., Tai, E., Batten, J. C., Hutchcroft, B. J. and Pepys, J. (1970) Cystic fibrosis—Immunological reactions to *A. fumigatus* and common allergens. *Clin. Allergy*, **1**, 1.
9. McFarlane, H., Holzel, A., Brenchley, P., Allan, J. D., Wallwork, J. C. and Singer, B. E. (1975) Immune complexes in patients with cystic fibrosis. *Br. Med. J.*, **I**, 423.
10. Shakib, F., Stanworth, D. R., Smalley, C. A. and Brown, G. A. (1976) Elevated serum IgG 4 levels in cystic fibrosis patients. *Clin. Allergy*, **6**, 237.
11. McFarlane, H., Allan, J. D. and Zeil, C. der (1977) Passive cutaneous anaphylaxis (PCA) and specific IgE in cystic fibrosis and their heterozygotes. *Clin. Allergy*, **7**, 279.
12. Warner, J. O. (1975) Atopy and cystic fibrosis. In: *Abstracts of the 6th Ann. Mtg. European Working Group on Cystic Fibrosis, Dublin, Ireland.*
13. Taylor, B., Norman, A. P., Orgel, H. A., Stokes, C. R., Turner, M. W. and Soothill, J. F. (1973) Transient IgA deficiency and pathogenesis of infantile atopy. *Lancet*, **II**, 111.
14. Wallwork, J. C. and McFarlane, H. (1976) The SIgA system and hypersensitivity in patients with cystic fibrosis. *Clin. Allergy*, **6**, 349.

CHAPTER 13

Allergy and the Nervous System

THE SIGNIFICANCE OF immunological mechanisms in diseases of the nervous system remains unsettled.[1] Allergic reactions occur following vaccinations, as a part of serum sickness and in association with some infectious diseases. There is some evidence that allergic mechanisms may also operate in other neurological and mental disorders such as convulsions, recurrent headaches (migraine) and behaviour abnormalities.[2-11,18,19] However, objective supportive data are few and much of the evidence is anecdotal.

It has been suggested that allergic reactions may occur within the hypothalmus and lead to the release of kallikreins which block the synthesis of nor-adrenaline, dopamine and serotonin, i.e. synaptic transmitters which have been implicated in some of the behaviour disorders. Some foods, food additives and chemicals are known to be potent activators of kallikreins.

Indirect evidence of the importance of allergic factors in causing neurological disturbances is available. For instance, in a group of 60 children with seizure disorders, EEG changes were observed in 73 per cent of the 37 allergic children and 10 per cent of the 23 non-atopic children. The use of elimination diets controlled seizures in 24 children and in whom the EEG changes either returned to normal or considerably improved.[5] Similarly, a study of 45 hyperactive children suggested that dietary control improved behaviour in 36 (80 per cent) children. The majority (75 per cent) of these children had other atopic conditions, e.g. rhinitis, eczema.[8]

Attacks of migraine can be precipitated by some foods such as cheese, chocolate or coffee. Undoubtedly tyramine in cheese and chocolate may be responsible and coffee may act by releasing catecholamines.[12,13,17] In an interesting study of 296 patients with thrombocytopoenia, 20 developed migraine-like headaches or classical migraine during episodes of bruising and low platelet count. Suggestion was made that the attacks were related to the changes in serotonin metabolism which in turn depends on the platelet activity since it is the major reservoir of serotonin in the blood.[14] There is also evidence that some migraine individuals have increased IgG levels and plasma from migraine subjects can produce abnormal release of 5-hydroxytryptamine from normal platelets.[15,16]

Clearly much remains to be learned about the possible role of allergy in causing nervous system disorders. It is my practice to try an elimination diet trial provided there is a convincing history, the child is atopic and the parents fully understand that such an approach to management is highly speculative.

References

1. Ridley, A. (1971) Clinical significance of immunopathological mechanisms in diseases of the nervous system. *Clin. Allergy*, **1**, 311.
2. Balyeat, R. M. and Rinkel, H. J. (1931) Allergic migraine in children. *Am. J. Dis. Child.*, **43**, 1126.
3. Glasser, J. (1954) Migraine in pediatric practice. *Am. J. Dis. Child.*, **88**, 92.
4. Hilsinger, R. L. (1974) Allergic headaches. *Otolaryngol. Clin. N. Am.*, **7**, 789.
5. Dees, S. C. (1954) Neurologic allergy in childhood. *Pediatr. Clin. N. Am.*, **1**, 1017.
6. Fowler, W. M., Heimlich, E. M., Walter, R. D., Smith, R. E., Grossman, H. J. and Helmy, J. (1962) Electroencephalographic patterns in children with allergic convulsion and behaviour disorders. *Am. Allergy*, **20**, 1.
7. Berman, B. A., Engel, G. L. and Glasser, J. (1959) The electroencephalogram in allergic children. *Am. Allergy*, **17**, 188.
8. Schneider, W. F. (1975) Psychiatric evaluation of the hyperkinetic child. *J. Pediatr.*, **26**, 559.
9. Campbell, M. B. (1973) Neurological manifestations of allergic disease. *Rev. Allergy*, **31**, 485.
10. Rowe, A. H. (1959) Allergic toxaemia and fatigue. *Am. Allergy*, **17**, 9.
11. Kittler, F. J. (1970) The role of allergic factors in the child with minimal brain dysfunction. *Am. Allergy*, **29**, 203.
12. Brown, J. K. (1977) Migraine and migraine equivalents in children. *Dev. med. Child Neurol.*, **19**, 683.
13. Ulett, G. A. and Perry, S. G. (1975) Cytoxic testing and leucocyte increase as an index to food sensitivity—II. Coffee and tobacco. *Annls Allergy*, **34**, 150.
14. Damasio, H. and Beck, D. (1978) Migraine, thrombocytopaenia and serotonin metabolism. *Lancet*, **I**, 240.
15. Mackarness, R. (1976) *Not All in the Mind.* London: Pan.
16. Anthony, M. and Lance, J. W. (1975) *Modern Topics in Migraine.* Ed. by Pearce, J., p. 107. London: Macmillan.
17. Editorial (1975) Headaches and coffee. *Br. med. J.*, **II**, 284.
18. Hall, J. (1976) Allergy of the nervous system: a review. *Annls Allergy*, **36**, 49.
19. Finn, R. and Cohen, H. N. (1978) 'Food allergy': Fact or fiction? *Lancet*, **I**, 426.

Index

Acetycholine 41, 52
Acrodermatitis enteropathica 47
Acrokeratotic poikiloderma 46
ACTH
  in asthma 108
  test 108
Adenoids
  and allergy 8
  and surgery 10, 80–81
Adrenal suppression 51
Adrenaline 61, 103, 121
Agammaglobulinaemia 46
Ahistidinaemia 46
Allergen extracts and immunotherapy
  76–78
Allergoids 75
Allergy 1
  and acute bronchiolitis in infancy 10
  causes 15–19
  incidence 3, 4, 7
  miscellaneous 9, 19
  physical agents 19
  risks of new allergies 4, 8, 10
Alphalactalbumin 17
Alpha-1-antitrypsin deficiency 24, 102
Anaphylactoid purpura 58
Anaphylaxis 1
  and drugs 126–127
  pathogenesis 127
  treatment 127–128
Angiitis, acute cutaneous 129
Angioedema
  diagnosis 55, 59
  hereditary 59
  treatment 59
Anhidrotic ectodermal dysplasia 46
Animal ephithelium tests 15

Antihistamines
  otitis media 88–89
  rhinitis 72
  skin diseases 60
Aspergillus fumigatus 17, 96, 99, 103
Aspirin sensitivity 8, 80
Asthma
  allergic factors 94, 95
  complications 103
  definition 91
  diagnosis 97, 102
  and exercise 100
  IgE (serum) 95–96
  incidence 91
  lung function 99–100
  mechanisms of 94–95
  mortality 91–92
  pathology 92–93
  physiology 92, 94–95
  prognosis 92
  tests
    provocation 98
    RAST 99
    skin 97
    specific precipitating antibodies 99
  treatment
    of acute attack 103
    with bronchodilators 106
    with corticosteroids 105, 107–108
    immunotherapy 108–111
    with sodium cromoglycate 107
    of status asthmaticus 104–105
  Type I reactions 96
  Type III reactions 97
Astrup formula for correction of
    metabolic acidosis 105
Ataxia-telangiectasia 46

Atopic dermatitis
  antihistamines 51
  clinical features 41–42, 44–45
  corticosteroids 50, 51
  diagnosis 45
  immunisations 49
  immunology 43–44
  immunotherapy 49–50
  incidence 42
  psychological factors 49
  treatment 47–52
  sodium cromoglycate 52
  miscellaneous 61
Atopy 1
Atropine and asthma 94

Bathing and skin 48–49
Beclomethasone dipropionate
    107–108
Betalactalbumin 17
Betamethasone valerate 107–108
Bicarbonate, sodium 105
Biopsy, intestinal
  in cow's milk 31, 35
Blood and allergy 30
Blood gases 106
Bloom's s. 47
Bradykinin 41, 52
Breast feeding and allergy 4, 5
Breathing exercises 111
Bronchial provocation tests 96
Bronchiectasis and asthma 103
Bronchiolitis, acute
  and allergy 10
Bronchitis, wheezy 30

Candida albicans (*see* thrush)
Casein 34
Cat dander 16
Cataract in atopic dermatitis 45
Charcot–Leyden crystals 93
Chest deformities in asthma 97
Chlamydia eye infections 115
Chocolate and headache 28
Chromosome anomalies and skin 47
Cobner phenomenon 57
Cockayne's s. (*see* ichtyosis)
Compliance, lung 95
Conjunctivitis
  allergic 114, 115–116

causes 114
  inclusion 115
  treatment 116–117
Contact dermatitis
  allergic 52–55
  irritant 52
  treatment 54–55
Contactants 18
Cor pulmonale 103
Cortical hyperostosis, infantile 30
Corticosteroids, adrenal
  in asthma 107–108
  in eye conditions 116, 117
  in rhinitis 73–74
  in skin disorders 60
  intranasal 74
Cosmetics 53
Cot death 30
Cotton lint 17
Cow's milk
  clinical features 15, 34
  diagnosis 31, 34
  and eyes 114
  pathogenesis 33, 34
  and skin 30
  treatment 35–36
Cradle cap 44
Cross reactions 15
Curschmann's spirals 93
Cyclic AMP 52
Cystic fibrosis and allergy 24, 134

Darier's sign 26, 58
Deafness 87
Dehydration in status asthmaticus 105
Delayed blanched phenomenon 43
Dennie's lines 25
Dermatitis (*see* atopic dermatitis)
Dermatographism 26, 43
Dermatophagoides pteronyssinus
  (*see* house dust mite)
Desensitisation, nasal 78–79
Diet 22
  elimination 32–33, 48
Dog dander 16
Dopamine and CNS allergy 136
Drug allergy 7–8
  clinical features 124–125
  diagnosis 131

prevention 131
treatment 127—128
Dubowitz s. and skin 47

Ear
allergy of
atopic dermatitis 86
contact dermatitis 86
serous otitis media
diagnosis 86—88
treatment 88—89
inner
Meniere's d. 89
Eczema
atopic 9
nummular 42, 45, 51
vaccinatum 9
Egg sensitivity 18
Environment and allergy 21
Eosinophils and allergy 47
Eosinophil chaemotactic factor 41, 52
Erythema
marginatum 58
multiforme 58, 128
nodosum 129
Eyes, allergy of
and drugs 7—8
examination 25, 115
immunology 114
management 116—117
Examination of allergic child 24—26
Exercise test in asthma 100—101

Face
in allergy 24—25, 70
Family history and allergy 22
Feathers 16
Fish allergy 18
Fixed drug eruptions 129
Flaxseed 17
Fluids in status asthmaticus 104
Food and allergy
allergens 17, 18
clinical features 29—30
diagnosis 30, 31
diet 32, 48
heredity 7
IgE 29
IgG 29, 56, 80
IgM 29, 56, 80
incidence 5—7, 27

neurological aspects 30, 136—137
pathogenesis 28
PRIST 32
RAST 32
skin tests 31
symptoms 29
treatment 32
Food intolerance 6
Food reactions, adverse 28
Functional residual capacity 100
Fungi (*see* moulds)

Games, effects of 22
Gastritis varioliformis 35
Gastrointestinal allergy 5—6, 23, 33—36
Genetics and allergy 6—8, 34, 42
Glaucoma and eye allergy 115
Gluten-induced enteropathy 47
Glycoproteins 18
Goblet cells 93
Granulomatous d., chronic, (Job's s.) 46
Grass pollens 15

Hapten 125—126
Hartnup's d. 46
Hay fever (*see* rhinitis)
Heiner's s. 30
Heredity 6, 8, 34
Histamine 41, 52
Histiocytosis-X 47
History 21—26
House dust 15, 109
House dust mite 15, 109
Humidification of room 48
Hygiene and skin 47
Hypersensitiveness 1
Hypersensitivity reactions
Type I 2, 29, 34, 56, 68, 95, 120
Type II 2
Type III 2, 29, 34, 96
Type IV 2—3, 29, 34
Hyperventilation 93, 94
Hypnotherapy 110—111
Hyposensitisation
(*see* immunotherapy)
Hypoxaemia in status a. 96, 104

Ichthyosis 46, 51
IgA and allergy 5, 56

IgD 29
IgE and allergy 1, 8
   in allergic rhinitis 10
   in atopic dermatitis 43, 47
   correlation with other tests 8, 99
   diagnosis 8, 29
   in psoriasis 7
   RAST 99–100
   in secretions 7, 80, 87
   serum 95
   in urticaria 8
IgG 6, 7, 29
IgM 6, 7, 29
Immunisations 30–31, 49, 111
Immunotherapy
   in asthma 108–111
   effects of 78
   indications 76
   insect stings 121–122
   mechanisms of 75–76
   methods 75
   in rhinitis 74–78
   in skin disorders 60–61
Incidence of allergic disease 7
Infections 94
Ingestants 17, 18
Inhalant allergy 15–16
Injectants 18
Insecticides 71
Insect allergy
   bites 119–120
   diagnosis 120–121
   stings 19, 119–120
   treatment 121–122

Kallikrein 136
Kapok 17
Keratoconus 45
Kidneys and drug allergy 30
Kinins 29

Lability index in asthma 101–102
Lanolin and allergy 44
Lavage, bronchial
   in asthma 106
Leiner's d. 46
Lungs and drug allergy 30
Lung function tests
   assessment 99–100
   diagnosis 100

response to treatment 102
Lyell's s. (toxic epidermal necrolysis)
   129
Lymphokines 28

Mast cell
   in allergy 35
   effects of drugs on 36
Mastocytosis (see urticaria pigmentosa)
Mediators 41, 52
Melkersson–Rosental s. 58
Meniere's d. 89
Methacholine 94
Methylxanthines 9, 103, 106–107
Migraine 7, 136
Milk allergy (see cow's milk)
Milk proteins 5–6
Moulds 17
Mucopolysaccharidosis 46
Mucus
   glands 93
   secretions 93
Myringotomy 87

Nasal tests
   diagnosis 99
   immunotherapy 78
Natural history of allergy 8
Nebulised bronchodilators 105
Nephritis and allergy 30
Nervous system and allergy 136–137
Netherton s. (see ichtyosis)

Orris root 17
Otitis (see under ear)
Oxygen in asthma 105

Paraben 53
Particles, allergens 15–16
Passive transfer test 93
Patch test in contact dermatitis 53–54
Pathology
   and asthma 92–93
   ear disorders 86
   eye conditions 114
   rhinitis 68
   skin disease 43
   others 88
Peak expiratory flow rate
   in assessment 98–99

in asthma 98
in diagnosis 98, 99–100
in exercise 100–101
in response to treatment 102
Penicillin allergy 125–126
Phenylketonuria and contact
    dermatitis 46
Photoallergy 55
Physiology
of asthma 94–95
Physiotherapy
in asthma 106
Pneumothorax 103
Pollen grains 15, 16
Polycythaemia, compensatory,
    in asthma 103
Polyps, nasal 80
Postural drainage in asthma 106
Precipitins, serum 99
Prevalence of allergy (see incidence)
Prognosis of allergy 8–11
Prostaglandins 8, 41, 52
Provocation test in asthma 98–99
Psoriasis 7
Psychological factor
in asthma 109–110
skin 49
Pulmonary eosinophilia 96, 103

Rabbit fur 16
Radioallergosorbent test (RAST)
in diagnosis 32, 99
principle and method 99–100
Radiology
in asthma 102–103
in rhinitis 71
Reaginic antibody 1, 28
Respiratory allergy 30
Respiratory failure in asthma 106
Rhinitis
causes 67
diagnosis 69–70
immunology 68
immunotherapy 74–79
incidence 68
investigations 70–71
surgery 80–81
treatment 71–81
Ritter's d. 45

Salbutamol 105
Schonlein–Henoch s. (see anaphylac-
    toid purpura)
School attendance and asthma 22
Secretory immunoglobulins 29, 56, 80
Serum sickness 130
Sinusitis 71
Sjogren–Larson s. (see ichtyosis)
Skin allergy (see also a. dermatitis)
causes 41–44, 128–129
clinical features 41–45
diagnosis 45
genetics 43–44
immunoglobulins 44
incidence 7
local applications 47–52
management 47–52
Slow reacting substance of
    anaphylaxis 29
Sodium cromoglycate (SCG)
pharmacology 35
uses in
    allergic conjunctivitis 117
    allergic rhinitis 72–73, 74
    gastrointestinal allergy 35–36
Status asthmaticus 104–105
Steroid aerosols 107–108
Stevens–Johnson s. 128
Sweating and skin allergy 43
Sympathomimetic agents 106
Symptoms, of allergy 21–24

Tar, coal or Lassar's paste,
    use of 51
Tension-fatigue s. 30, 136–137
Terbutaline 103
Tetracosactrin test 51
Theophylline (see also
    methylaxanthines)
action of 103
blood levels 106–107
uses of 9, 106
Thrush, oropharyngeal 74, 108
Tomato allergy 18
Tonsillectomy and allergy 10
Toxic epidermal necrolysis
    (see Lyell's s.) 129
Trantas spots 116
Twins and allergy 2
Tyramine and headache 28

Ulcerative colitis 33
Ultraviolet light and skin 55
Urticaria
    causes 55
    clinical features 56–57
    diagnosis 58–59
    immunology 55–56
    incidence 55–56
    pathogenesis 55
    treatment 59–61
Urticaria pigmentosa (mastocytosis) 58

Vaccination and allergy 9
Vegetable allergy 18

Ventilation–perfusion in asthma 92–93
Virus infections 45

Weather conditions 48
Wheat allergy 87
Whole body plethysmography 100
Wiskott–Aldrich s. 7, 46
Wool sensitivity 17, 18

Xanthines (*see* methylxanthines)
X-rays (*see* radiology)

Yeast (*see* thrush)